W9-BZD-645

"Sick of the scale being the boss of me, I needed a different voice in my head. Then I stumbled upon Wendy's 40-Day Sugar Fast, and suddenly the spiritual connection between food, my heart, and God clicked for me. I started to see food as less of a reward or a temptation and more of a means to align my heart back with God's. Food, like all of His good gifts, should always point us back to the Giver. It shouldn't accuse us or guilt us. It should simply remind us what we need to sustain us. This shift in thinking has taken me forty days and beyond. And I'm so grateful for the mental overhaul more than any pounds lost. More than anything I want to be able to say with Jesus, 'My food is to do the will of him who sent me' (John 4:34). And traveling with Wendy and the 40-Day Sugar Fast community was the beginning of that journey for me."

Lisa-Jo Baker, bestselling author of *Meet Me in the Middle*,
Never Unfriended, and *Surprised by Motherhood*

"If Wendy is leading, I want to follow. This woman is exceptionally wise with an impressive earnestness for leading people to the feet of Jesus. She is a highly respected mentor and communicator with a passion for pointing people to what matters most. Wendy is much more than a writer who can string a bunch of nice words on the page. Her words bring real results."

Jennifer Dukes Lee, author of *The Happiness Dare* and *Love Idol*

"We all want freedom. We want to break free from habits that haunt us, voices that taunt us, chains that bind us, and emotions that blind us. Wendy's onto something huge here! She speaks with depth and authority from the Word of God, and she knows that the emancipation we're all really longing for is actually a person: Jesus. *The 40-Day Sugar Fast* helps each participant experience meaningful growth and lasting peace, as it ushers them to a fresh, personal, and satisfying banquet with the One who longs to be their portion."

Gwen Smith, cofounder of Girlfriends in God and author of
I Want It All and *Broken into Beautiful*

"To fast from what we crave in order to find sustaining satisfaction in God is a message for this clamoring culture. And it's a message for me. Wendy's words are for every one of us whose reach for sugar is never enough."

Sara Hagerty, bestselling author of *Unseen*

"Each day of Wendy Speake's book *The 40-Day Sugar Fast* shifted my cravings for sweets to the sweet words of Jesus. I couldn't have broken the stronghold of sugar without Wendy's gracious and wise influence in every chapter. A life-changing book to be read over and over again!"

Amber Lia, bestselling coauthor of *Triggers* and *Parenting Scripts*

"Too many Christian women today feel trapped by sugar cravings and addiction, wondering if they'll ever break free. Through her annual 40-Day Sugar Fast, Wendy has offered thousands of women, myself included, the opportunity to taste the sweetness of Jesus and experience His bondage-breaking power in their lives. Truly, freedom and fullness are found only in Jesus's presence, and Wendy has proven herself a worthy guide year after year."

Asheritah Ciuciu, author of *Full*

"I have to share a praise report. I believe that my addiction to sugar is gone for good! I can't believe it's been two years since I last fasted with Wendy and my cravings are not back. God really changed my perspective about sugar and food during those forty days. I did this fast three years in a row, but that time there was real and lasting change! I'm reminded of how Elijah kept going back and looking for rain, and finally he saw a little cloud and then the rain!"

Amy J. Bennett, founder of Abiding Ministries and host of the podcast *Feathers*

"Wendy Speake is gifted at capturing biblical truth in profoundly relevant ways to help us discover new ways of thinking about not only sugar and our addiction to it but also the strongholds that keep us from experiencing the fullness of God's presence in our lives. If you're ready to fast from sugar so that you can feast on more of God's Word, *The 40-Day Sugar Fast* is for you."

Elisa Pulliam, biblical transformation and wellness coach at MoreToBe.com and ItIsWell.us

40-Day Sugar Fast Testimonials

"Every day for forty days, I said, *Jesus, I need You. You are enough.* That prayer changed my life."

Chanda T., CA

"I am teary just thinking of where I am now compared to forty days ago. I am twenty-nine pounds lighter, my skin and mind are clearer, and (most importantly) I am closer to my one true love, Jesus. He was so good to me during this fast. I have never been able to resist sugar before. And yet, I have not missed it. Oh how He loves me!"

Lynn K., MA

"It's been years since I've gone more than three days without chocolate. I knew this fast was something I needed to do. Chocolate made days doable. Now, I'm learning Jesus makes days doable. And livable. And abundantly full."

Kristin G., TN

"Fasting has unlocked so many doors inside my heart that were closed off for far too long. I have a long way to go with some of the things God has revealed, but for the first time, I feel equipped. I feel ready to put on the full armor, step out onto the battlefield, and fight the good fight. Thank you, Wendy."

Barbara N., MI

"Over these forty days it has been refreshing to not run to sweets every time something went wrong. Since I didn't run to sweets first, Bible verses came to mind when I needed them—at the most appropriate times, in a way I hadn't experienced before. God faithfully showed me that He has been there waiting for me to simply seek Him. I feel like this is just the beginning—I feel that God broke strongholds I've lived with for so many years."

Beth I., CA

"Day 40 of this sugar fast is not the end for me! I have hope and faith that when this is all over, because I have fed on Jesus, I will not ever revert back to my old ways."

Hannah S., Australia

"What an absolute blessing this fast has been for me. I'm sugar FREE!"

Ronda M., CA

"This sugar fast is a direct answer to prayer!"

Anne Marie L., CA

"This has been an amazing journey. The thing I'm most grateful for is that I am walking away with a more intense desire to let Jesus fill my cravings with His Word and not relying on my sweet tooth."

Kyla N., PA

"I fought God so much about my sugar, coffee, TV, and social media . . . yet I've given them up and I don't miss them because I have found true satisfaction in Him. My prayer these forty days has been, *Lord, I don't want to go back to the same person I used to be. I want to continue to know You more, daily. I need You to satisfy my soul.*"

Kris D., TX

"God has been so present these forty days. I am beyond grateful. He has been so alive in me and has taken another sin-struggle and helped me through. I could never have done this on my own. I am going to continue feasting on the Lord!"

Michelle O., MI

"I admit that I originally wanted to do the 40-Day Sugar Fast to streamline my dieting process. However, I quickly learned God had so much more in store for me. He called me to Himself in ways I've never experienced before. I get fasting now. I didn't before. I understand why God calls us to it and asks us to rid ourselves of physical desires so we can turn our hearts to Him."

Megan S., CO

"Amazing! I felt led to do the 40-Day Sugar Fast because I needed to quit sugar. Little did I know all the transformation that God had in store for me."

Ashley T., FL

"My skin is less wrinkled and broken out. My stomach has flattened a bit. But internally, I finally feel at peace. I'm not chasing all the things. And it feels so good."

Jaymie M., IL

"I came to this sugar fast specifically as a way to intercede for my family. First, I asked God to heal my two-year-old son, so that he can live without a feeding tube. Second, I needed God to redeem my marriage. Here's the praise: halfway through this fast, my son was taken off the feeding tube, and by the end of the fast, he was gaining weight. And my husband and I are in a good place together! My tummy is a little empty, but my heart is so full!"

Whitnee M., AR

THE 40-DAY

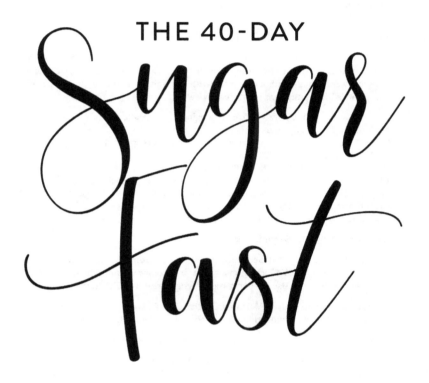

WHERE PHYSICAL DETOX MEETS
SPIRITUAL TRANSFORMATION

WENDY SPEAKE

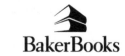

BakerBooks

a division of Baker Publishing Group
Grand Rapids, Michigan

Published by Baker Books
a division of Baker Publishing Group
PO Box 6287, Grand Rapids, MI 49516-6287
www.bakerbooks.com

Printed in the United States of America

Library of Congress Cataloging-in-Publication Data
Names: Speake, Wendy, 1974– author.
Title: The 40-day sugar fast : where physical detox meets spiritual transformation / Wendy Speake.
Description: Grand Rapids : Baker Books, 2019.
Identifiers: LCCN 2019017286 | ISBN 9780801094576 (paperback)
Subjects: LCSH: Sugar-free diet. | Detoxification (Health) | Food—Sugar content.
Classification: LCC RM237.85 S67 2019 | DDC 613.2/8332—dc23
LC record available at https://lccn.loc.gov/2019017286

ISBN 978-1-5409-0111-8 (hardcover)

The Author is represented by the William K Jensen Literary Agency.

To the women who joined me online for the first sugar fast five years ago—I didn't feel equipped to lead, still you followed me as I followed Jesus. He's brought us a long way since then! Our diets have changed but our lives have changed even more. This book is dedicated to you and to the One we followed together in those first forty days.

Open your mouth and taste,
open your eyes and see—how good GOD is.
Blessed are you who run to him.

Psalm 34:8 MSG

Contents

Foreword   11

Before You Fast   15

Guidelines   21

DAY 1   Taste and See   27

DAY 2   Return to Me   32

DAY 3   When Sugar Walls Crumble   37

DAY 4   Trusting God with the Battle   42

DAY 5   Fasting and Feasting   47

DAY 6   Armor Up!   51

DAY 7   A Holy Hunger   56

DAY 8   Candy Canes and Crutches   60

DAY 9   When Jesus Shares His Food   64

DAY 10   His Presence, Our Present   68

DAY 11   Shine!   73

DAY 12   Food Triggers   77

DAY 13   Weight and Worship   82

DAY 14   What Else Are You Craving?   87

DAY 15   Divisive Devices   92

DAY 16   Comfort Foods and Retail Therapy   97

DAY 17   Be Quiet and Be Transformed   101

DAY 18   Stumbling Blocks and Dynamite   105

DAY 19   Have a Sober Mind   109

DAY 20   The World's Goods Aren't as Good   113

DAY 21   Boredom Can Be a Trigger Too   118

DAY 22   Spiritual and Mental Clarity   122

DAY 23   Hunger Pangs   126

DAY 24   Healing Past Hurts   130

DAY 25   God Cares about the Details   136

DAY 26   As for Me and My House . . .   140

DAY 27   The Kind of Fasting God Wants   145

DAY 28   Feed My Sheep   150

DAY 29   Ditto   155

DAY 30   At the Table with Jesus   159

DAY 31   Praying for Healing   163

DAY 32   Wake Up!   168

DAY 33   Brick by Brick   172

DAY 34   Remember!   176

DAY 35   Once You're Free, You're Free to Share   180

DAY 36   Two Masters   184

DAY 37   Keep Knocking, Keep Asking   188

DAY 38   Getting Down to the Root   193

DAY 39   God Wants Your Life, Not Your Sugar   198

DAY 40   Live Like It's True!   203

DAY 41   He's Not Done with You Yet   207

Appendix A: Life beyond the Fast   211

Appendix B: Additional Resources   215

Acknowledgments   217

Notes   219

Foreword

DO YOU LOVE ME MORE THAN SUGAR?

That thought startled me out of my reverie. What kind of a question was that?! Of course I loved Jesus. I grew up in church, surrendered my life to Him at the age of five, and have faithfully served Him ever since. I have loved Jesus as far back as I can remember.

But if you'd have to give up sugar—for the rest of your life—would you do it? This new thought threw me. Now why would I do that?

Would you choose Jesus over sugar? The questions pelted me like an unwelcome hailstorm.

This was getting out of hand. Of course I'd choose Jesus. I'd given my life to Jesus! I'd die for Him!

Then why are you running to cookies instead of running to the cross? Why do you seek solace in a pint of ice cream rather than the Prince of Peace? Why are you feasting on warm bread rolls instead of the Bread of Life?

Ouch.

My life slowly came into focus, scenes from past binges flashed before me. I slowly realized that with my mouth I confessed one thing as true, but my eating habits revealed another truth entirely.

Sugar was my savior, not Jesus.

My heart broke in two.

"What do I do?" I cried out to the empty sunroom. The sunbeams streamed through billowy curtains as despair overran my soul. My eyes fell to the paragraph I had underlined just moments before those daunting questions first came to my mind. This time I read more slowly.

> If you don't feel strong desires for the manifestation of the glory of God, it is not because you have drunk deeply and are satisfied. It is because you have nibbled so long at the table of the world. Your soul is stuffed with small things, and there is no room for the great. God did not create you for this. There is an appetite for God. And it can be awakened. I invite you to turn from the dulling effects of food and the dangers of idolatry, and to say with some simple fast: "This much, O God, I want you."[1]

This much, oh God. This much.

. . . As much as I crave my morning mocha.

. . . As much as I desire a second serving of pie.

. . . As much as I anticipate the taste of my next sugar fix.

That much? No. If I was being honest, I didn't desire God that much. But I wanted to.

"Help me want You more," I wrote in my journal that day. "Stir in me a hunger for You." That's when the Spirit began piercing my soul with His convicting questions, not to heap condemnation but to lead to inner transformation. His invitation to me was clear: a forty-day fast from sugar to break the stronghold it had become in my life and train my affection on Christ alone.

I drew in a shaky breath and agreed.

A few days into my sugar fast, withdrawal hit me hard. What had I done? What was I thinking? This was crazy! Not only had my sugar cravings intensified but a hidden part of me had surfaced that I had never seen before. I was irritable, impatient, and intent on getting my way. I snapped at anyone who so much as looked at me the wrong way.

All I could think about was sugar: donuts, milkshakes, creamer, cookies, instant oatmeal . . . even ketchup. Sugar was everywhere, and I was craving it with reckless abandon, much like a drug addict. The pull toward sweets seemed magnetic.

"I'm not going to make it," I confessed under my breath when a coworker brought cookies to share at work. "I can't do this anymore."

But God, being rich in mercy, provided just what I needed. I learned that an online friend was leading a sugar fast—oh the "coincidences" that come when we learn to trust Him!—and I immediately signed up to join her, eager for the community and accountability.

Wendy proved a trustworthy companion. Gentle yet firm, she redirected my gaze away from my momentary sacrifice to fix my eyes on the grand prize. Not skinnier thighs or a healthier thyroid, not glowing skin or grounded emotions. No. These may have occurred, but my reward was Jesus.

Jesus.

He is enough. And in fasting from the small things of this world, like sugar, we invite Him to awaken in us a hunger for Him. "He satisfies the longing soul, and the hungry soul he fills with good things" (Psalm 107:9)—yes, even with Himself.

Those forty days with Wendy taught me that I didn't really have a sugar issue after all—I had a heart issue. Jesus wants our undivided, unadulterated affection. He wants us to love Him with all our hearts, all our souls, all our minds, and all our strength (Mark 12:30). All of us. Everything. Every last molecule crying out for more of Him. And when we beg Jesus to lead us to that place of longing, He will gladly satisfy us with the very best He has to offer—Himself.

The enemy of our souls comes only to steal, kill, and destroy, and he often uses sugar addiction to cripple us spiritually, emotionally, and physically. But Jesus has overcome, and He offers us the full life found in Him alone (John 10:10).

That first fast became the battleground where I discovered the truths I share in my book *Full: Food, Jesus, and the Battle for Satisfaction*. Over the years that followed, Wendy graciously invited me to join her in leading the 40-Day Sugar Fast, and together we have seen thousands of women encounter the freedom and fullness found in Jesus when we give Him everything—even our sugar addiction.

This journey will not be easy, friends, but it is so worth it because Jesus is our satisfaction and He is our reward.

Better even than chocolate cake?

Oh, yes. Come and see.

Asheritah Ciuciu, author of *Full: Food, Jesus, and the Battle for Satisfaction*

Before You Fast

"MY NAME IS WENDY AND I'M A SUGAR ADDICT."
Those nine little words changed the trajectory of my life when I posted them online in 2014. Innocently, I invited people on my Facebook page to join me for a 40-Day Sugar Fast. I wasn't simply having a problem with sugar, I told my friends, I was experiencing physical and emotional problems too. My sugar tooth was dictating my thoughts and my days. On top of that, constant neck pain and stomachaches plagued me. I was gaining weight, my muscles and joints were always hurting, my sleep was fitful, and my emotions were a wreck. I was grumpy, tired, and impatient with my kids and my husband. Sadly, sugar wasn't making me sweet. I didn't need any more conviction, what I needed was transformation. I needed more than another diet; I needed something deep within me to change.

The response to my online invitation was overwhelming. "Me too," they cried. "Yes!" they affirmed. "My name is Melissa . . . My name is Alexis . . . My name is John . . . My name is Jenn . . . and I'm a sugar addict." There's something about sugar that has a grip on us, and we know it. We run to sugar for our comfort and our reward. We turn to it in boredom. We depend on it when life is stressful. We crave it when we're depressed and use it as confectionary therapy. And even when life is at its best, we celebrate with cake.

We've been running to sweet snacks to get us through our days for far too long. It's become a habit. No, worse than that, it's become an *addiction*. And addiction works much like a prison. We're unable to break out of the bars and the bondage that hold us back from health and wholeness. Men and women the world over have traded their freedom—along with their health—for sugary shackles, and they're so ashamed.

If that's you, if you are feeling powerless over your addiction to sugar, if you have lost sight of God's power in your life, know that you are not beyond redemption. **Fad diets and workout routines can't set you free, but God can.** Sugar is everywhere but so is He. What would you be willing to give up in order to gain the powerful presence of God in your life? With His help you can be set free—free from your shame, free from your cravings, free from your addiction.

> *Fasting is merely denying yourself something temporal and ordinary in order to experience the One who is eternally extraordinary.*

Join me for this forty-day journey to food freedom, faith, and the discovery that He is enough. Lay down sugar so that you might taste and see His good and satisfying sweetness in your life. Fasting is merely denying yourself something temporal and ordinary in order to experience the One who is eternally extraordinary.

What This Book Is and Is Not

Before you turn another page, let me clarify what this book is and what it is not. It isn't a scientific source recounting the evils of sugar; there are plenty of books that do that. Nor is this a diet book or a collection of recipes. While I love to cook and share some of my favorite meals with others, I am not a nutritionist. I am simply a Jesus-hungry woman who is passionate about turning hungry hearts toward the only One who can ever truly satisfy.

Are you a binge eater? A secret eater? An emotional eater? Tell the Lord all the reasons why you can't go forty days without sugar, and let Him show you that with Him it's possible (Matt. 19:26). Over the course of these next few weeks, as you stop cramming food and other fillers into the hurts and holes of your life, the power of Christ will fill each empty place with His peace. He will make you whole.

Nutritionists and diet experts encourage us to "crowd out sugar" by eating plenty of delicious and nutritious foods. I love that idea and have used the same technique in my own eating habits. However, the purpose of the 40-Day Sugar Fast isn't just physical detox; the goal is spiritual transformation. Not only will we be fasting from sugary sweets, we'll also be fasting from all the things we turn to instead of Him. The 40-Day Sugar Fast is primarily a spiritual fast, so the main way we will "crowd out sugar" is by intentionally turning to the Lord and consuming His living Word instead. We are focusing on taking in more of Him and less of the things that don't make us more like Him.

We suffer spiritually each time we reach for a sugar high rather than the Most High. Our sugar fixation stops us from fixing our eyes on Jesus, and hungering for sweet treats gets in the way of our hunger and thirst for Him. **The goal of this fast isn't that you will begin to choose healthy food options; it's that you will come to see Christ as the only option.** The more you ingest of Him, the less hungry you will be for the things you once craved. **We're fasting from sugar so that we might feast now. This is how we crowd the sugar out.**

Think of this book as a daily companion to help you do just that. Each day's reading is packed with Scripture and application so that you might feast on God's Word in lieu of the world's sweetest fare. Ingesting sugar might not make us sweet but consuming Him certainly does. Sweet and satisfied and stable. Physically, spiritually, and emotionally so.

We're fasting from sugar so that we might feast now. This is how we crowd the sugar out.

If you want His peace, love, joy, and gentleness, and you're desperate for His self-control, turn to Him. Abide with Him. He's told us clearly, "Those who remain in me, and I in them, will produce much fruit. For apart from me you can do nothing" (John 15:5 NLT).

The 40-Day Sugar Fast is for those who are sugar-dependent but long to be dependent on God. You've tried to muscle through and grab hold of self-control—and all the other fruits of God's Spirit—on your own, but it doesn't work that way. **Abide in Him, consume Him, and His fruit will consume you and transform you.**

How to Begin

Perhaps you're convinced that this fast is what you need, but you don't know where to begin or what to expect. I understand. But don't worry, it's quite simple.

Make a commitment to join me in saying no to refined sugars for forty days. No sugary snacks, baked goods, ice cream treats, sweet coffee creamers, sodas, candies, and so on. Nothing that includes refined sugar or high-fructose corn syrup. From there, the specifics are up to you. Some people choose to avoid all forms of sugar, while others use limited amounts of raw honey, maple syrup, and fresh fruit in their diets. Some keep Stevia, Erythritol, and monk fruit on hand, while others feel convicted to lay all sweeteners down during the fast. Many say no to the sneaky sugars hidden in marinades and condiments such as barbecue sauce, teriyaki sauce, and ketchup, but others don't. Plenty of people cut all simple carbs from their diet as well, along with alcohol and anything else that turns to sugar in the gut. You'll need to make some choices before you begin.

Take a day or two to pray before you fast. Ask God to show you what your fast should look like. You're not putting on a show for anyone else. Privately seek His will for your private fast. What will work best for you and your family may be different from what will work for me and my family. **Ask God to speak to you about anything in your kitchen that you're running to in a frenzied or habitual attempt to satisfy your soul's deep hunger and then give it to Him as an offering.** Maybe He will lead you to simply stop eating donuts, drinking mochas, and grabbing an afternoon Snickers bar and late night bowl of ice cream. Or perhaps He will speak to you about the alcohol in your cupboard that not only turns to sugar but can easily become a daily reward that you run to as soon as it's five o'clock somewhere.

Seek Him first before you fast. Tuck this Scripture-promise deep in your heart and frame it on your kitchen counter: "But seek first the kingdom of God and his righteousness, and all these things will be added to you" (Matt. 6:33).

Seek Him daily as you fast, filling yourself with more of Him and His righteousness, and you will likely drop pounds. But that is just a by-product of something weightier still. While your weight may decrease, your faith will increase and God's power will begin to flow in your life again. **Fasting from physical food increases one's spiritual hunger, and that's the hunger that** leads not only to a transformed body but also to a transformed life. When we empty ourselves and ask Him to fill us, He does. When we are at our weakest, His strength is most evident. When we don't know what we're doing, He does it all. **When God sets us free from the strongholds in our lives, we're free to experience His strong hold.**

I'm excited to journey through the next forty days with you. Let's kick this sugar fast off with a prayer, because communicating with God is what turns this physical fast into a spiritual one.

Dear Lord, nothing has worked to set me free from the compulsive way I turn to sugar when I could be turning to You. Before I even begin this fast, I know I need more of You and less of the stuff that leaves me hungry. Take all the refined sugars I'm laying down and teach me to lean into Your gentle refining. Take my life as I empty it out and fill me with Yourself. Your Word proclaims: "It is for freedom that Christ has set you free." I'm choosing to believe that's true. Set me free! In the bondage-breaking, freedom-giving, sweet, sweet name of Jesus, Amen.

Guidelines

YOU HAVE MADE A COMMITMENT to say no to all your sugary sweet treats for the next forty days. Nothing made with sugar. No soda or syrupy drinks. No ice cream, donuts, pancakes, cake, or Peanut M&M's. Nothing containing sugar or high-fructose corn syrup. Beyond that, it's between you and the Lord. Take the details of this fast to Him in prayer. Should you keep fresh fruit in your diet? How about natural sweeteners such as raw honey and maple syrup? Since breads and pastas are broken down into glucose by your body and cause an increase in blood-sugar levels, many people choose to fast from them as well. Talk it through with the Lord, and make a plan before you fast.

What You Can Eat

Before you fill your heart, you have to empty your heart of what has been filling it. The same is true in your kitchen.

This book doesn't focus on what you can eat because the goal of this fast is that you increase your devotion to God—not your devotion to sugar-free foods. Rather than substituting one treat for another, allow yourself to go hungry. Treat yourself to more of God in lieu of food. You are fasting so that you might learn to feast on Him. **Don't simply switch your obsession with sugar for a sugar-free obsession—obsess over the One who** cares more about transforming your life than transforming your diet.

I realize that you may need a little practical help as you prepare your pantry, stock your fridge, and learn to prep meals as you fast and pray. Here are some ideas to get you started.

1. *Take a moment to remove all the high-in-sugar and highly processed items in your pantry and refrigerator.* Simply bag them up and hide them from sight. Better yet, give them away. It may feel like you're throwing away money but think of it as trashing temptation.

   Don't forget your special stash of chocolate. Our favorite sweets are often the hardest to toss. Start there. Don't put them in the freezer to keep, put them in the trash to lose. It's possible that when you finish forty days of fasting from sugar, your whole outlook on what you eat and how you eat and why you eat will have changed. If you go back to the old treats on day 41, you'll find yourself right back where you started. **Toss the temptation before you're tempted.**

2. *Stock your pantry and fridge with healthy food options.* Here are some of my favorite foods to keep on hand as I fast from sugar.

   Pantry:
   Raw nuts
   Nut butters
   Unsweetened, dried fruit
   Unsweetened coconut flakes
   Chia, flax, and sunflower seeds
   Dehydrated veggie chips
   Lara or RX bars

Beef sticks and beef jerky

Oatmeal and sugar-free granola

Olive oil, avocado oil, coconut oil, and ghee

Balsamic vinegar, rice vinegar, and apple cider
vinegar

Salt, pepper, herbes de Provence, and other spices to
keep veggies and meats tasting good (and not the
same night after night)

Fridge:

Precooked rotisserie chicken

Plenty of poultry, fish, and beef

Sandwich meat and cheese

Eggs (hard boil a few)

Seasonal vegetables (leafy green lettuce such as
spinach and kale, eggplants, broccoli, asparagus,
brussels sprouts, tomatoes, cauliflower, and
squash)

Seasonal fruits in moderation (raspberries, strawber-
ries, blueberries, kiwis, lemons, grapefruit, green
apples, grapefruit, and watermelon)

Avocadoes

Hummus

Pesto

Sparkling water and herbal tea

3. *Take the time to do some meal planning.* I like to prep a
couple of large batches of my favorite meals each week
so that I'm not obsessing about food as I fast. This isn't
the time to become the world's best sugar-free cook.
You want to keep your focus on fasting from sugar, not

transfer your focus to sugar-free cooking. **Keep it simple so that you can see that He is simply enough.** Here are a few (simple) favorites I like to keep on hand.

Chili and soups

Taco meat to add to salads

Chicken salad (which is easy to take on the go)

Large egg dish for a quick high-protein breakfast or snack

Find a few of my favorite recipes at 40daysugarfast.com.

4. *Avoid using sugar substitutes.* While I keep raw honey and Stevia on hand when I need to sweeten something for a family meal, I purposefully choose not to make sugar-free desserts when I fast from sugar. I hope that you will join me. We don't want to exchange our high-calorie addictions for sugar-free options; instead, we should grow to desperately crave Jesus as the only option. Remember, this fast is yours. Take the details to the Lord and ask Him to guide and convict you as you make your plan.

5. *Choose which day you will begin and then invite your family and friends to come along.* While fasting is a very private thing, accountability increases when you invite others to come into the intimate space of your prayer closet with you. You've welcomed guests around your table and served them the sweetest food you've had to share, but this experience is sweeter still. You'll be surprised how many of your family members and friends say yes to joining you!

ADDITIONAL RESOURCES

If you would like additional books to help you meal plan or better understand what is happening with you physiologically or spiritually as you fast and pray, check out appendix B at the back of the book for a list of suggested resources.

day 1

TASTE AND SEE

Taste and see that the Lord is good;
  blessed is the one who takes refuge in him.
Fear the Lord, you his holy people,
  for those who fear him lack nothing.
The lions may grow weak and hungry,
  but those who seek the Lord lack no good thing.

Psalm 34:8–10 NIV

WHEN I WAS A YOUNG CHILD, I was all about the sugar. I craved candy with every fiber of my being. It was sweet and it was good and it was an exciting part of my weekly routine. Every Friday after school I got two dollars for my allowance, immediately hopped on my little pink bike—the kind with the white wicker basket—and pedaled to the corner store a few blocks away. My neighborhood friend Kerry had an equally impressive sweet tooth, so I'd swing by her house first. Together we'd go fill that basket with Cherry Bombs and Lemon Drops, strawberry Nerds, peach Jelly Bellies, sour apple Jolly Ranchers, Red Vines, and Reese's Peanut Butter Cups.

Walking into that corner store each week, the bell over the door announcing our arrival, was a happy ritual for me. Just thinking about it reminds me of the scents and makes my mouth water. I can even feel the thin, soft crinkle of the brown paper bag that the elderly Japanese man who owned the store put my candy into. I also remember how generous he was with the pennies he kept in an ashtray beside the register. If my purchase was ninety-one cents, he would take a penny from the dish and put it in the register with my dollar bill and hand me back a dime. Kerry and I would step out into the bright afternoon sunlight, jump on our bikes, and ride the cracked sidewalk back to one of our houses. Oh how we loved our sugar!

On the afternoons when I didn't have a nickel to my name, I would come home from school and scour the back of the refrigerator where my mom often hid the half-emptied tub of Betty Crocker's vanilla frosting. As I sat watching *Little House on the Prairie*, one spoonful from the tub would turn to two, then three, then four, until the tub was empty.

Since both of my parents worked, I had a key dangling from a shoestring around my neck. As a latchkey kid, I had plenty of time home alone to make some unhealthy habits for myself. Don't get me wrong; I'm not blaming my parents for my sugar addiction. There are plenty of kids who learned to stash their sugar in the bottom drawer of their desks, under lined paper and a collection of heart-shaped erasers, with Mom and Dad just down the hall.

Why am I sharing this with you? Because I need to remember where I came from and how I got here. You do too. The treats we loved and the memories we have tied to them have led many of us here today. We have loved our sweets for a long time, but we are finally ready to love God more. Though our sugar has been a faithful friend to us, we are eager to forge a new friendship with a faithful God, a God who promises to make things new for us. We're ready to build new memories—memories of turning to Him when we're happy and running to Him when we're sad. We've been running to the wrong things for far too long.

Perhaps you've read the Bible, and believed the promise that God is good, but how much better it will be to actually taste and see His goodness for yourself. That's the transformation we're after. However, it is absolutely possible to read the Bible, fast and pray, feel convicted, and still choose to remain unchanged. Transformation isn't automatic—you have to put God's Word into practice.

I know because that same little girl who rode her bike to the corner store on Friday would also sit in a pew on Sunday. Here's what I've discovered: Sunday morning messages don't always influence the everyday habits of our lives. We're told that God alone can save us, that He alone can satisfy us, that we can taste and see His sweetness and ingest Him as our daily bread . . . but then we hop on our metaphorical little pink bikes and pedal our way to the store or to anything else that promises to fill our baskets, our hearts, and our lives.

It is absolutely possible to read the Bible, fast and pray, feel convicted, and still choose to remain unchanged.

What have you been running to? That's the type of question I'm learning to ask myself as the Sunday service comes to a close. As the worship team plays one more song and the congregation begins to leave, I ask myself, *Where am I pedaling off to these days? What am I running after? If all this is true, how should my life look? If Jesus truly came to set me free, why am I still running to food? If I really have been bought with a price . . . If Jesus fasted and prayed and literally fed His disciples . . . If Jesus alone can satisfy my deepest longings . . . If . . . If . . . If . . .*

If what I learn on Sunday mornings is true, it should affect everything about how I spend my days: the way I love my family, the way I hold my thoughts captive, the way I spend my money, the food I eat, the words I say, and all the details of my life. Everything that I do needs to line up with God's Word.

Psalm 34:8–10 is a passage I pray over and over when I am fasting.

> Taste and see that the LORD is good;
> blessed is the one who takes refuge in him.
> Fear the LORD, you his holy people,
> for those who fear him lack nothing.
> The lions may grow weak and hungry,
> but those who seek the LORD lack no good thing. (NIV)

We are no longer children, friends. The One we worship on Sunday must remain Lord over our lives Monday through Saturday. We are mature men and women who have been invited by the Lord Himself to taste and see how good He is all week long. He has invited us to run to Him when we're tempted to run into the corner store (whether grabbing candy or a bottle of wine). We can run to Him rather than running to the recesses of our pantry. And we can run to Him and find refuge in Him when we're tempted to hide behind our phones.

The One we worship on Sunday must remain Lord over our lives Monday through Saturday.

His invitation calls us out of all our habits and immature addictions, whether we're abusing sugar or bingeing on Netflix shows and YouTube videos. God calls out to each of us, "Taste and see Me. Hide yourself in Me. Let Me be what you run to! All other beasts suffer hunger, even the lion. But not humanity. No, I have redeemed humanity for

Myself, and those who come to Me, who taste and see Me for themselves, will lack no good thing."

Dear Lord, I have a long history with sugar. You know I do. You were there as my habits were formed. But those years are behind me now. My future with You, however, stretches on forever. Please help me to make You my new habit. Help me run to You so that I might taste Your sweetness and allow You to satisfy all my needs. In Jesus's satisfying name, Amen.

day 2

RETURN TO ME

"Even now," declares the LORD, "return to me with all your
heart, with fasting and weeping and mourning."

Joel 2:12 NIV

I REMEMBER THE FIRST DAY of my first 40-Day Sugar
Fast. I came to it with great hope of experiencing joy in God's
presence. I had three young boys and I was worn out and joy-
less. As I entered into that season of fasting, I quoted Psalm
16:11 expectantly: "In your presence there is fullness of joy."
Yes, I was after joy and eager to be filled to overflowing. I don't
think there was anything wrong with that prayer. After all, it
is biblical. Scripture tells us that when we abide with God, we
will bear the fruit of His joy in our lives (John 15:5). Fasting is
abiding on a gut level—an *empty* gut level.

When I stopped filling my emptiness with sweet treats so
that I might be filled up with God, His Spirit surprised me.
Before God led me up to the high places of gladness, He took
me through a valley of deep sadness. He flooded my heart with
conviction, and conviction felt more like heartache than happiness. As I realized how far I'd drifted from God's presence,

I experienced a holy sort of sadness. No wonder I was hungry for joy; I'd wandered from the Joy Giver. Before I could be satisfied by His joy-inducing presence, I had to grieve over how far I'd strayed, and return to Him. "'Even now,' declares the LORD, 'return to me with all your heart, with fasting and weeping and mourning'" (Joel 2:12 NIV).

Fasting is abiding on a gut level—an empty gut level.

Here on the second day of your sugar fast, I invite you to take an honest look at where you are and where God is in relation to you. He is not a far-off God; He hasn't gone anywhere but it's possible that you have. It may be that instead of running to Him to fill you, you have been running to the pantry. Perhaps, instead of opening up your Bible, you've been opening up your smartphone and scrolling through social media. It's not sugar, but it is another filler.

What do you turn to instead of to Him? Take a few moments today to consider this question. If you find that you habitually turn to anything but Him, I urge you to deal with your wandering prayerfully and to seek Him faithfully. Weep, mourn—and return to Him for in His presence you will find the joy you've been searching for.

I'm reminded of the Christmas story and of the name Jesus was given before His birth. Matthew 1:23 proclaims the angel's message: "'Behold, the virgin shall conceive and bear a son, and they shall call his name Immanuel' (which means, God with us)." The name *Immanuel* proclaims Jesus's mission: to be with us. And, by His indwelling Holy Spirit, Jesus remains a very near and present God. Unfortunately, our free will allows us to wander from the One who promised never to wander from us. So today, we need to purpose in our hearts (and in our lifestyles too) to turn back to Him—to return.

The Old Testament is full of stories about the waywardness of God's people. Their unfaithfulness broke the hearts
of many of the prophets and biblical leaders. Joel, Jeremiah,
Isaiah, Ezra, and Nehemiah all fasted, praying that God would
turn the hearts of His people back to Him.

Take a moment to read Nehemiah's prayer below.

> LORD, the God of heaven, the great and awesome God, who
> keeps his covenant of love with those who love him and keep
> his commandments, let your ear be attentive and your eyes
> open to hear the prayer your servant is praying before you day
> and night for your servants, the people of Israel. I confess the
> sins we Israelites, including myself and my father's family, have
> committed against you. We have acted very wickedly toward
> you. We have not obeyed the commands, decrees and laws you
> gave your servant Moses.
>
> Remember the instruction you gave your servant Moses, say-
> ing, "If you are unfaithful, I will scatter you among the nations,
> **but if you return to me and obey my commands, then even if
> your exiled people are at the farthest horizon, I will gather
> them** from there and bring them to the place I have chosen
> as a dwelling for my Name." (Neh. 1:5–9 NIV, emphasis mine)

Allow Nehemiah's prayer to inspire one of your own. Pick up
a pen and write out a prayer of repentance (or lift up your voice
and cry out). Ask the Lord to help you see your own wayward
tendencies, and then confess them. He is faithful to forgive you
and welcome you back into a restored relationship with Himself
because of His Son, our very present Savior.

Throughout the Scriptures and throughout history, people
have struggled to remain in God's presence. Time and again we
wander away only to feel the pain of putting distance between
ourselves and the Father. If that is where you find yourself

today, weep and mourn and return to Him. It is my experience that once you return to the Joy Giver, joy isn't far behind.

So consider this: Is it possible that you have wandered away from God? Perhaps you know it's true, but you aren't sure what it would look like to turn from your old ways or if you even can. You've experienced conviction but don't know how to get to transformation. You know your tendency to fashion a makeshift god

It is my experience that once you return to the Joy Giver, joy isn't far behind.

from sweet confectioneries but you haven't been able to stop. Pinpoint your vices and repent—turn around, pull a complete 180, and go in the opposite direction. If you've been running to all the wrong fillers in lieu of the only One who can fill you up and make you full, repent. Confess it to the Lord "with fasting and weeping and mourning." Turn and return to Him.

Dear Lord, thank You for being my Father, even when I am a wayward child. I'm sorry. Your forgiveness is life! And because I've been so completely forgiven time and time again, I ask that You bind me close to Your heart and help to keep me in step with Your joy-giving Spirit. In Jesus's name, Amen.

SOME THINGS TO BE AWARE OF WHILE YOU FAST

Your body is detoxing as you fast. That physiological reality is likely intensifying your emotions as well. While I believe that fasting heightens your spiritual senses, causing conviction and repentance, I know that cutting out sugar cold turkey can cause emotions of sadness and anger to flare up as well. In the early days of your fast, you may experience what many refer to as a "sugar flu." As you go without your tasty mood enhancers, you may feel grumpy or emotional. This is normal and common when you first embark on a sugar fast. You've been dependent on sugar for far too long, and that's partly why you feel miserable without it. Let your awareness of your dependency on sugar rather than on Christ convict you of your waywardness and prompt you to turn and return to Him. And as you do, be on the lookout for joy. While sugar provides a temporary jolt of happiness, this promise is long and lasting: "Weeping may last through the night, but joy comes with the morning" (Ps. 30:5 NLT).

day 3

WHEN SUGAR WALLS CRUMBLE

As soon as the people heard the sound of the trumpet, the people shouted a great shout, and the wall fell down flat.

Joshua 6:20

SUGAR IS A STRONGHOLD for many people. Does it hold you back from the good life that God has planned for you? Perhaps over time your sweet tooth has turned into a full-fledged addiction, dictating your days, driving you from one sugary fix to the next. **Unfortunately, no sugar fix can fix you.** In fact, when you give sugar that job, you'll end up more broken than before because sugar weakens our physical bodies and clouds our minds. If only you could break free from this sweet, strangling stronghold, but you feel powerless. The walls are too thick and too wide, the habits too ingrained, the enemy too big and too strong, and you are too addicted.

However, all throughout the Scriptures, God demonstrates that He has the power to open prison gates and set captives free. Today I encourage you to shout God's victory over your life even before He helps you tear down the stronghold of sugar. Why? Because that is exactly what God instructed the Israelites to do as they marched around the strong walls of the city of Jericho. This massive stronghold was in their way, preventing them from entering God's promised land. For the walls to come tumbling down, God's people had to first shout the victory. In full obedience and faithful expectancy, they lifted up their voices to Him in praise.

Do you know the story? Did you sing the song about Joshua and the battle of Jericho when you were young? Do you know that the same power to bring down strongholds is available to you? We read in the book of Joshua, chapters 5 and 6, that Joshua was taking Israel from their wilderness wandering into the promised land. But before they could take possession of God's good promises, they had to pass through Jericho. The city walls were high and well-fortified, and the people of Israel felt hopeless.

That's when a man with a drawn sword appeared to Joshua, saying he was the commander of the Lord's army. Joshua fell down in reverence at his feet. The warrior told him to remove his sandals for he was standing on holy ground, and then the Lord spoke to Joshua, telling him exactly what he needed to do. For six days all the mighty men of war were to march around the walls of Jericho one time. Behind them the priests would follow, blowing on rams' horns. On the seventh day, however, they were to march around Jericho's walls seven times, with the priests blowing their horns continually. After the seventh time around the stronghold, the Lord commanded all the people of Israel to shout triumphantly. Then and only then, would the walls come tumbling down.

What a thrilling story! If you've never read it for yourself, please take a moment to ingest it now. It is my hope that you see that the Bible is so much more than a thrilling story; it's your story and mine. My fasting friend, just as the fortified city of Jericho was blocking the Israelites from entering the promised land, the stronghold of sugar may be holding you back from the abundant life God has planned for you. For that reason, I encourage you, amid your withdrawal symptoms and cravings, to give praise to the Lord because of what He's *about to do*. Shatter the strong hold sugar has on you and replace it with a sweet dependence on Him.

The same God who set His people free from bondage in Egypt, the same God who parted the Red Sea and led them across dry land, the same God who fed them in the wilderness and delivered them from their enemies and finally ushered them into the promised land is alive and available today.

> *The same God who saves also speaks! So listen.*

Here are five takeaways from the crumbled walls of Jericho that can help you on your journey from slavery to freedom.

1. **Believe that this place is holy (Josh. 5:15).** If you want the Lord to do a deep soul-work in you, slip off your shoes and place the soles of your feet on holy ground. God is at work in you and you get to march, barefoot and believing, through these forty days. Plant your feet on the solid ground of faith.

2. **Ask Him to tell you His plan for you (Josh. 3–7).** God gave the Israelites specific instructions about how to take down the stronghold of Jericho. He will do the same for you if you ask Him for help with each challenge you face.

   This wasn't the only time God gave His people clear directives. He spoke to Esther as she fasted and prayed,

He spoke to Daniel as he fasted and prayed, He spoke to King Jehoshaphat as He fasted and prayed. The details of each fast were different. The circumstances of each life were different. The questions were different. And God's answers were all uniquely different. God will give specific instructions that apply to your circumstances as you fast and pray. Ask Him what His plan is for you.

3. **Listen to the Lord (Josh. 6:2).** God is not a far-off or silent being. He has given you His living and active Word, along with His living and breathing Spirit, to be in communication with his people. **The same God who saves also speaks! So listen.** Allow the Lord who spoke clearly and kindly to Joshua to speak directly to your heart. Though His Word is inspired for all, He whispers to individuals in a private and loving manner. In order to hear Him, you must get quiet and listen.

> *God, what walls do You want to bring down?* Listen.
> *What does freedom in You look like?* Listen.
> *Is there anything else that You want me to fast from?* Listen.
> *How do I do this?* Listen.
> *When should I meet with You and pray each day?* Listen.
> *What's Your plan for me as I fast?* Listen.

4. **Obey (Josh. 6:8).** The old hymn says it best, "Trust and obey, for there's no other way to be happy in Jesus but to trust and obey."[1] Fasting requires obedience. And extended fasts like this one will require extended obedience. It's easy to justify changing things up a bit mid-fast in order to make it easier. I know from experience. However, when you stay committed to doing what God

has told you to do (I'm talking following God's clear leading, not legalism), God in His supernatural power enables you to bring down the strongholds in your life. Yes, even the stronghold of sugar. The people of Israel had to march for seven days before they experienced deliverance. You have committed to forty days. Keep marching in obedience.

5. **Shout the victory before the walls fall (Josh. 6:20).** This is your main charge today. Shout His praise, believing in what He *will* do before He even does it. The same God who has set captives free can set you free today. Believe Him and shout His victory over your dependence on sugar.

God, You are strong and good and faithful. I'm shouting Your praise before a single brick falls from the walls holding me in and holding me back. You are able to set me free from all addictions, to heal all hurts and get to the root of what's causing my sin and sadness. I can't stop praising You for what You have already done in my life. I am confident that You will bring down the strongholds in these present struggles. Lord, You are able and You are God. I'm blowing my horn and shouting Your name. Amen.

day 4

TRUSTING GOD
WITH THE BATTLE

Listen, King Jehoshaphat and all who live in Judah and Jerusalem! This is what the LORD says to you: "Do not be afraid or
discouraged because of this vast army. For the battle is not
yours, but God's."

2 Chronicles 20:15 NIV

THE FIRST YEAR I hosted the 40-Day Sugar Fast online I
posted a picture of an old vinyl record on our private Facebook
page and asked my friends to help me put together a playlist of
songs we could sing at the start of our fast. Hundreds of people
responded in the comment thread with links to their favorite
praise songs. We had worship music to last us forty days and
well beyond! Ever since that first year, compiling a list of worship songs has become an annual tradition at the start of each
of our community fasts because, when we sing songs of worship, we proclaim out loud that the battle belongs to the Lord.

Four days into this fast, your body may feel like it is going
through a physical battle. Perhaps you feel like the fast is your

enemy or that sugar is your enemy or that your children are your enemy or that I am your enemy. Today I want you to focus on letting go of the fight and embrace praise, trusting that God will go to battle on your behalf.

I'd like to share a story from the Bible about a man who faced a terrible battle. In 2 Chronicles 20:1–30, Jehoshaphat, king of Judah, received word that "a great multitude" was advancing against him. "Jehoshaphat was afraid and set his face to seek the LORD, and proclaimed a fast throughout all Judah. And Judah assembled to seek help from the LORD; from all the cities of Judah they came to seek the LORD" (vv. 3–4).

When we sing songs of worship, we proclaim out loud that the battle belongs to the Lord.

The first thing that strikes me about Jehoshaphat is that he was *afraid*, yet he sought God's help. Perhaps that's where you are right now: afraid of the withdrawal symptoms, afraid of laying down your addiction, afraid because you've already cheated on this fast and wonder if you should just give up, afraid of failing further . . . If so, I encourage you to take a moment to set your face toward the Lord. You've intentionally turned your eyes away from food, but have you decidedly turned your eyes to God in sugar's stead? Are you seeking His help as you fight this battle?

Read these words from Psalm 121:1–2 with me.

> I lift up my eyes to the mountains—
> where does my help come from?
> My help comes from the LORD,
> the Maker of heaven and earth. (NIV)

King Jehoshaphat came from the lineage of David, the man who wrote the lyrics to the psalm-song above. David penned

Psalm 121 as he hid from his enemy, King Saul. Similarly, these words from Psalm 56:3–4 came to him when he was captured by the Philistines: "When I am afraid, I put my trust in you. In God, whose word I praise, in God I trust; I shall not be afraid. What can [man] do to me?" What a picture both David and Jehoshaphat paint for us. When they were afraid, they turned to God.

You've intentionally turned your eyes away from food, but have you decidedly turned your eyes to God in sugar's stead?

Jehoshaphat, however, didn't do it alone; he asked his people to fast and pray with him. Can you imagine all the people of Judah, fasting and seeking God together? I'm reminded of this promise from Psalm 33:12: "Blessed is the nation whose God is the LORD, the people he chose for his inheritance" (NIV).

Jehoshaphat believed this and invited his people to believe it too. Together they fasted and together they prayed, and consequently God came to their aid, told them what to do, and assured them of victory.

> Listen, King Jehoshaphat and all who live in Judah and Jerusalem! This is what the LORD says to you: "Do not be afraid or discouraged because of this vast army. For the battle is not yours, but God's. Tomorrow march down against them. . . . You will not have to fight this battle. Take up your positions; stand firm and see the deliverance the LORD will give you, Judah and Jerusalem. Do not be afraid; do not be discouraged. Go out to face them tomorrow, and the LORD will be with you." (2 Chron. 20:15–17 NIV)

Immediately, Jehoshaphat fell on his face and worshiped. And all the people of Judah followed him to their knees. Every one of them laid prostrate before God. That's when some of the Levites—Israel's worship leaders—stood and sang praises in a very loud voice. "As they began to sing and praise, the LORD set ambushes against the men of Ammon and Moab and Mount Seir who were invading Judah, and they were defeated" (v. 22 NIV). The priests sang, and God Himself defeated their enemies as Jehoshaphat and his men looked on.

God assured King Jehoshaphat and the Israelite people that He would deliver them, and so they celebrated their victory *before* God defeated their enemies. Yesterday we learned that God's people shouted before the walls tumbled; today we see that they sang before an army tumbled. They believed that the battle belonged to the Lord. Do you? Are you muscling through the early days of this fast on your own or are you singing your faith songs out loud, trusting that this battle belongs to Him?

God is still speaking this same message over you now with His promise: "Do not be afraid or discouraged because of the battle you face today [where food or anything else is concerned]. The battle is not yours but mine." Therefore, go out today with praise on your lips and your eyes fixed on Him.

Mighty God of angel armies, thank You for giving me the story of King Jehoshaphat to grow my faith today. When he was afraid, he knew where to turn. I have turned to other gods in my fear, my loneliness, my emptiness, and my pride, to give me courage and strength each day. But the battles of this life continue to rage, and I need You, Redeemer. Only You. I choose to set my face toward You today. As I wait to see You move, I will sing Your praises and eagerly anticipate Your deliverance. In Jesus's name, Amen.

YOUR SWEETEST NEMESIS

Speaking of going to battle, sometimes sugar feels like the enemy. Agreed? The average American eats between 150 to 170 pounds of refined sugar every year.[1] While that may seem impossible at first glance, the reality is that it's not hard to accomplish. Four sodas a day times 365 days a year amounts to nearly 150 pounds of sugar! Oftentimes during our online sugar fasts, I hear from men and women who discovered that sugary treats in general isn't their problem, their problem is Dr Pepper . . . their problem is sweet tea . . . their problem is wine . . .

Take a moment to pinpoint your "enemy." What's your sweetest nemesis?

day 5

FASTING AND FEASTING

> Your words were found, and I ate them,
> and your words became to me a joy
> and the delight of my heart.
>
> Jeremiah 15:16

A FEW DAYS into my last fast, I was putting dishes away when I noticed two of our family Bibles on the kitchen counter. My husband's big, blue study Bible and the slender, brown, leather-bound one I usually keep in my purse. As my stomach growled, I found myself inspired. Immediately I pulled out my prettiest cake stand and placed it on the countertop, stacking the Bibles on it. Together they looked like a multitiered cake on display. I smiled.

Over the next thirty-five days, I kept the cake stand front and center as a reminder. When I found myself bored and looking for something to nibble on, I was reminded to feast on the Word! Each time I was tempted to mindlessly grab a handful of sugar-coated something, I'd grab hold of my well-worn Bible instead. Fasting from sugar and feasting on God's words became the theme of my afternoons and evenings—any time of the day or night that my stomach growled again.

The imagery of consuming God's Word is found over and over throughout Scripture. In Ezekiel 3:3 we read that God fed the prophet Ezekiel a scroll containing His Words. God said to Ezekiel, "Son of man, eat this scroll I am giving you and fill your stomach with it." To which the prophet responded, "So I ate it, and it tasted as sweet as honey in my mouth" (NIV).

In Revelation 10:8–11, John was charged to eat the scroll that an angel handed to him. Devouring God's Word is the secret to our fasting days, the key to stopping us from consuming anything and everything else. As I mentioned in the introduction, we are crowding out sugar with the satisfying sweetness of Christ, and the main way we are doing that is by ingesting His Word.

Are you hungry to ingest the transforming and filling presence of Christ? You get to do that each time you "consume" His words. When you read John 6, for example, you eat up the story of Jesus feeding the five thousand and believe that He can fill you in miraculous ways. Then you read on and ingest the account of Him walking on water, and you're ready to jump out of the boat and follow Him too because you have tasted and seen Him for yourself.

Each time I fast from food, I rediscover that Christ truly is as sweet as honey in my mouth. Unfortunately, after some time has passed, the flavor fades and the things of this world attempt to crowd Him out again. That's why I fast for forty days *a few times each year*. It's not that I want to live a fasting life, it's that I need to live a feasting life. Each time I forget to feast, I fast in order to remember. Don't think of fasting as a magic trick. Abracadabra, once and done. Fasting may transform your diet, but it is a feasting life that will change your life.

> *Each time I forget to feast, I fast in order to remember.*

One of the practical things I've learned during my seasons of fasting and feasting is that God's Word can be served up all day long in different sized portions. There are snack-sized portions for on-the-go encouragement, main courses when we can really sit down and feast, and desserts that are sweet reminders of just how loved we are! The first time I led this fast online, my dear friend Christy Nueman sent me a long list of Bible passages and categorized them for me this way: "Here are some wonderful *snacks* for you, Wendy," she wrote before listing her favorite verses. "Enjoy these main courses," she prefaced a list of longer, meatier passages—many of them whole chapters. And then, under the heading "Desserts," she put some of the most familiar verses that are applicable when I needed a loving reminder of God's sweet presence and faithful promises.

Practically speaking, here's how I live out this feasting life. In the morning, when I wake up early enough, I snack on a verse or two to help me fix my eyes on a truth. I don't have much time to myself since I am often rushing my kids off to school, so I enjoy my main meal of the day once I have them all settled. I read an entire chapter, sometimes multiple chapters, and then write out the verse that the Lord used most mightily to speak to me. That verse becomes a snack-sized portion I take with me everywhere I go. Oftentimes I read it in a few translations on the Bible App and then link over to other verses that flesh the lesson out further. I write down one or two of those as well. If I struggle during the day, I reach for one of the familiar verses that I've loved for years and years as a midday dessert to remind my heart how loved I am. When I get a text from a friend in need of encouragement, I reach again for those verses and send them off like a care package. Often, the people I encounter each day need exactly what I've been feasting on.

Do you see what I mean? You must remain in the Word. Five minutes of nibbling on a verse in the morning won't fill you up and fuel you through the other 1,435 minutes of the day. You need a continual feast to carry you through long fasting days. First Thessalonians 5:17 tells you to "pray without ceasing." If praying is talking to God, then reading God's Word is listening. Let's make the *conversation* a continual feast! Read and pray, then read and pray some more. Let your fasting days propel you into a feasting life!

Five minutes of nibbling on a verse in the morning won't fill you up and fuel you through the other 1,435 minutes of the day.

Keep your Bible open on your kitchen counter, my fasting friend, on a cake stand or open on top of your recipe books. Write down the verses that you read—even the ones I've included here in this book. Write them out on an index card (or a recipe card) and carry them with you to snack on. Better yet, open up the Word and read the verses I share in the context of the chapter. That's the feasting life!

Sugar offers you empty calories, but Christ's Word is sustenance. It is the meat that sticks to your ribs and turns to spiritual muscle, so that you might be strong to live out what He tells you to do.

Oh Lord, You are so good to chase me down in the midst of my addictions and afflictions. This is about so much more than sugar. Teach me to live a feasting life as I spend these next few weeks fasting and praying continually. In the redemptive name of Jesus, Amen.

day 6

ARMOR UP!

Finally, be strong in the Lord and in the strength of his might.
Put on the whole armor of God, that you may be able to stand
against the schemes of the devil. For we do not wrestle against
flesh and blood, but against the rulers, against the authorities,
against the cosmic powers over this present darkness, against
the spiritual forces of evil in the heavenly places.

Ephesians 6:10–12

AS I BEGAN WRITING THIS BOOK, my computer started
autocorrecting *Holy Spirit* to *Hokey Spirit*. When I shared this
with one of the women who was fasting with me, she exclaimed,
"Get behind me, Siri!" which made us both laugh. Of course, she
was being punny, making a play on words out of Jesus's strong
command, "Get behind me, Satan" (Matt. 16:23). But even as we
laughed, I recognized that the devil had been working overtime
in my life since I began *The 40-Day Sugar Fast*. Perhaps you've
been experiencing something similar now that you're on this
journey from fasting to feasting.

**Satan hates you. But for the most part, he pays you no
mind as long as you are entangled in sin and struggling with**

shame. He likes you lethargic and ineffective. He prefers it when you struggle with migraines and emotional instability, when you are irritated with your spouse and your kids and your coworkers. He loves it when you blow up at your family or friends over a sugar-induced spike and crash. However, when you turn to Christ for His free and freeing power, Satan takes offense and goes on the offensive. He hates it when you fast and pray because he knows that each time you go to God rather than to sugar to fill your longings, the Spirit of God floods into the empty places in your heart and life. Satan hates losing ground.

When you started your forty-day fast from sugar, you may have anticipated temptation, but you may not have expected the tempter himself. The good news is that "the one who is in you is greater than the one who is in the world" (1 John 4:4 NIV). Each day, as you go to Him rather than to food, the Spirit of God gives you strength that those empty calories never could! As you turn to Him, He moves into your heart and into your home and into your neighborhood.

Each day, as you go to Him rather than to food, the Spirit of God gives you strength that those empty calories never could!

That is why as God advances, the devil advances right up into your intimate business. In fact, I don't doubt that as soon as you began fasting, you experienced at least one, if not many, of the following:

- conflict with friends
- a spike in negative self-talk
- financial challenges
- angry outbursts at your loved ones

- annoyance with your spouse
- misunderstandings with colleagues and neighbors

If so, be encouraged. Why? Because the devil is not happy that God is taking His rightful place at the center of your life. First Peter 5:8 says that the devil is prowling around like a roaring lion looking for someone to devour. When you were stuffing your face, comforting yourself with food instead of turning to the Comforter, the devil paid you no mind. Now that you're on the alert, however, Satan has been alerted!

Thankfully, God has written out exactly what you need to do in order to fight this spiritual battle and win. Ephesians 6:10–18 tells you to armor up! You're told to dress for battle every day, but I'm telling you to especially prepare as you fast and pray. Tie truth around your waist, and make it a double knot! Put on the protective breastplate of righteousness to guard your heart. Slip on your gospel-shoes and walk out your faith. Lift high your shield of faith, which is able to protect you from the devil's attacks. And wield the sword of the Spirit, which is the Word of God. Finally, put on the helmet of salvation.

While I hope that you'll meditate on all the spiritual armor at your disposal, I want to focus in on the helmet of salvation today. I believe that many, if not most, spiritual battles begin in the mind. This is especially true where addiction is concerned. That's why it is critical that you discipline your mind to think spiritually.

Years ago, I was working through a Bible study by Beth Moore. In it, Beth painted a picture with her words that has stayed with me. She asked us to imagine ourselves holding the helmet of salvation in our hands each morning, filled to the brim with the cleansing and protective blood of Christ. Then she said that when we lift it up and place it on our heads each new day, Christ's blood covers us anew—running down from the top of our heads to the bottoms of our gospel-loving feet! We're sealed from head to toe! But it all starts at the top, with our thinking. Begin each day of this fast by affirming:

> Whatever is true, whatever is noble, whatever is right, whatever is pure, whatever is lovely, whatever is admirable—if anything is excellent or praiseworthy—think about such things. (Phil. 4:8 NIV)

Here's what is true: If you have put your faith in Jesus Christ to save you, He has! And because you've been saved, God has the power to continue to save you today and tomorrow and throughout these forty days and beyond. Remember that. Remember what's true when the fiery darts fly. Your helmet of salvation is covering and protecting your mind today.

Before your feet hit the floor, remind yourself: "I've got an enemy and he wants my life today, but my life is safe in Jesus's hands." Focus your thoughts on what is true about God, even when Satan slithers in with his lies. Even when your life doesn't testify that God is good and protective and near, remind yourself that He is, has been, and will always be. Use your lips to declare, "My life and my thought life are completely bound up in Christ. He is for me. So, Satan, get behind me!" When the devil tries his best to stir up strife, speak aloud what you know to be true, and tell him to take a hike.

The same God who saved you eternally has the power to save you internally.

"I know what's true; I know who I am and whose I am . . . get out of here!" The same God who saved you eternally has the power to save you internally. Believing that truth is where the spiritual fight begins.

Place your thought life in His capable hands as you put on that helmet to guard your thinking today. He alone is able to save you from every weapon formed against you. I know it sounds allegorical, but you are in a literal battle. Satan would love nothing more than to keep you from your freedom in Christ, so armor up!

Dear Lord, thank You for keeping me in Your perfect peace when I actively fix my daily thoughts on You. Keep me steadfast and immovable, stayed and secure, believing what is true each day. Help me to prioritize putting on my armor at the start of each new day. This fast is not merely a physical detox but a spiritual battle, which is why I need You and Your full armor, Holy Spirit! In Jesus's name, Amen.

day 7

A HOLY HUNGER

Blessed are those who hunger and thirst for righteousness, for they shall be satisfied.

Matthew 5:6

AS YOUR BODY DETOXES in the weeks ahead, remember that no amount of sugar has *ever* been able to satisfy your hunger. Sugar's temporary pleasure is short-lived. Fleeting. Think about it. Even when you've just had a slice of key lime pie on a hot summer's day or a serving of apple cobbler in celebration of fall's bounty, don't you often hunger for more? I know I do, no matter the season. As I'm scraping food off of dinner plates and wrapping up leftovers to stick in the fridge, somehow I always end up eating "just one more bite." I had to go through this forty-day sugar fast three times—that's one hundred and twenty days without sugar!—before I began to understand my problem. **My issue isn't actually with sugar, or with food, but with hunger—misplaced, insatiable hunger.**

Now, it's true that there are physiological reasons why sugar is tremendously addictive. But there are deeply spiritual reasons too. Nothing convicts me of my sugar fixation quite like fasting does because when I stop running to sugar, I realize how my misplaced hunger has kept me from running to God. My hunger for sweet treats gets in the way of my hunger and thirst for Him.

Fasting from eating doesn't change our hunger, but when we exchange what we hunger for, it can change the way we eat.

Fasting from eating doesn't change our hunger, but when we exchange what we hunger for, it can change the way we eat. The only way I've learned to change my hunger is to change my mind about what I'm most hungry for.

In Christ's clear-spoken Sermon on the Mount, he said, "Blessed are those who hunger and thirst for righteousness, for they shall be satisfied" (Matt. 5:6). What does this mean in light of our insatiable appetites? If we want to live satisfied lives, we must focus on the One who is able to fill us with a reservoir of righteousness!

When we change our minds about what we're most hungry for, when we finally begin to hunger for His righteousness, our eating habits start to change, as do our lives. That's when we begin to be transformed. Here's how it works: As we feast more on the Word and less on food from the fridge, His Word transforms our minds. It changes how we think about life and God. Not only that, our bodies are also changing. Because we are eating less food, we are also losing weight and gaining more energy. I've said it before: The size of our waists will decrease as the size of our faith increases. We will become increasingly more interested in spending time with Him instead of running to the pantry or connecting with friends online. For when we start to crave the True Bread, we will be filled and fully satisfied.

It is my hope that you don't simply read a few verses and pray a few prayers and drop a few pounds during these forty days. If that's all you do, then the pounds will likely come right back, along with your insatiable appetite. Instead, I pray that you discover a different sort of hunger—a holy hunger that leads to a satisfied life.

I have a handful of friends who model this hungry, holy life. Even in busy seasons with young children and overwhelming work schedules, they take the time each morning to sit at Jesus's feet, hungry for His Word and His presence. He is their chief concern. Years ago, one of these friends told me that she has prayed a prayer inspired by Matthew 5:6 for the majority of her adult life: *Lord, help me to hunger and thirst for Your righteousness more than anything else.* Each time I go on a sugar fast, her simple Scripture-prayer comes to my mind and directs my own prayers. In the early days of your fast, I encourage you to pray it too. Exchange what can never satisfy you for the only thing that can. When we grow in our devotion to Him, we grow in our hunger for Him and His righteousness.

> *Exchange what can never satisfy you for the only thing that can.*

As the deer pants for streams of water,
so my soul pants for you, my God.
My soul thirsts for God, for the living God.
(Ps. 42:1–2 NIV)

My fasting friend, you've got to change your mind about what it is you're most hungry for today. It's been seven days since you started your sugar fast, and you are likely still experiencing some pretty intense cravings. Allow each one to bring you to your knees. Ask God to help you exchange your sweet tooth with a new hunger for the satisfying sweetness of Christ. When you hunger most for Him, it will change your life. Your hunger for sugar will decrease, and your hunger for Him will increase. This holy hunger will transform more than your diet; it will transform your life.

Dear Lord, as the deer longs for streams of water, so I long to long for You. For You alone can satisfy thirsty souls and fill hungry hearts with that which is good. Therefore, Lord, I'm asking You to help me with Your Spirit—help me to hunger and thirst for Your righteousness more than anything else. In Jesus's name I pray, Amen.

day 8

CANDY CANES AND CRUTCHES

Behold, God is my helper;
the Lord is the upholder of my life.

Psalm 54:4

I WAS IN HIGH SCHOOL the first time I heard an atheist argue that Christians are just weak people in need of a crutch.

"Jesus," he accused, "is the crutch you lean on to get you through this life." I was only sixteen years old, but I remember thinking, *Of course He's a crutch. Praise God for sending His Son for us to lean on, with the fullness of our fallen weight, or we'd be hobbling through this crazy life alone.*

I couldn't understand why this combative boy in my geometry class was challenging my faith with that ridiculous crutch analogy. The image of Jesus holding me up, making me able-bodied and sure-footed, only strengthened my believing heart. "You're right," I conceded, "you're absolutely right. Christians need Jesus every day. However, I think we're all leaning on something. But I've come to believe that whatever we lean on in this life better have the ability to get us ready for the next life too."

"Heaven?" he asked with a sneer.

"Leaning on Jesus in this life is the only thing that will allow us to walk into His eternal kingdom when this life is over. But put heaven aside if you want. We all need something to lean on. Perhaps you're leaning on your abilities just as heavily as I'm leaning on my Savior's ability to hold me up."

God is absolutely a crutch! He's the only crutch that enables us to not only walk through the valleys on this earth but also to run full-speed ahead into the high places of eternity. Praise the Lord for his sustaining, upholding, and eternal support.

The trouble is, sometimes I forget that faithful crutch and grab other things to get me through at three o'clock in the afternoon when the stresses of life add up. It's often in the midst of real life stress that I forget to lean on the real Life Giver. For instance, when my school-age kids are melting down over math homework and my husband has just called to say that he'll be late, I sometimes grab a handful of chocolate chips. When I've been cleaning the house all day but still have three loads of laundry to fold and put away, I have been known to throw some highly sugared creamer into my afternoon cup of coffee or tea. When I've had a challenging morning at work, I often grab a leftover brownie from the night before to push me over the hump. Instead of leaning on Christ, I lean on something fleeting to boost my adrenaline and give me a surge of dopamine so that I will feel better.

It's often in the midst of real life stress that I forget to lean on the real Life Giver.

Even as I write this, what comes to mind is the image of a candy cane, which is made to look like an actual cane or, better yet, a crutch. The problem with leaning too heavily on a candy crutch is, almost immediately, it breaks and I break too, because God never intended for sugar to sustain me. Instead, God says, "Cast your burden upon the LORD and He will sustain you; He will never allow the righteous to be shaken" (Ps. 55:22 NASB).

Big burdens, daily burdens, seemingly insignificant burdens. God can handle them all when you place them in the palm of His hands. Other translations of Psalm 55:22 similarily exhort, "Cast your cares upon the Lord . . ." I like that image too. You can cast your cares on Him because He cares for you.

You can cast your cares on Him because He cares for you.

In contrast, sugar doesn't give a rip about your joy or your health, your stress or your family, your ability to bear the fruit of God's Spirit in your life or your emotional well-being. My friend Amy Bennett journeyed with me through the first couple of sugar fasts, and one day she came to a profound conclusion. She likened her sugar addiction to an abusive relationship. By the end of one of our fasting seasons, she realized that she loves sugar, but sugar doesn't love her back. Like a hurtful, unbalanced suitor, over and over again, sugar showed Amy its inability to be faithful and loving. So Amy made the hard choice to break up with sugar, once and for all.

You're only one week into your fasting, but perhaps you see yourself in Amy's story. Believe me when I say that candy crutches can't hold your weight; they only increase it. Only Christ is able to hold you up. Because Jesus sacrificed His life, He alone is able to save and sustain yours.

Nowadays when I think of the crutch analogy, I imagine a cane—not a candy cane but a shepherd's staff. Jesus was the ultimate Good Shepherd and I am the epitome of a foolish, wayward sheep. But I know my Shepherd's voice, and I can hear Him calling me back into His presence again. Jesus is the true and faithful lover and sustainer of my soul. He leaves the ninety-nine to grab me each time I wander off. Jesus picks me up and carries me back with the full weight of my burdens resting on his shoulders.

Friends, all other crutches will break under the weight of your burdens. Only Jesus can pick you up and carry you today, because He alone has the authority and power and position to carry you into an eternal life with Him. So praise God for sending His Son so that you don't need to hobble through another day alone. Because of Jesus, you can run, full-speed ahead, into this abundant and eternal life! Lean your full weight on that.

Dear Jesus, I'm leaning on You today, as I lean into Your Word. You and You alone are able to make me able-bodied. You can carry my burdens because You care for me. You are able to sustain my life because You gave Yours. No one else and nothing else was created to carry my weight. Thank you, Jesus. It is in Your name I pray, Amen.

day 9

WHEN JESUS SHARES
HIS FOOD

"My food," said Jesus, "is to do the will of him who sent me to finish his work."

John 4:34 NIV

I LOVE EATING OUT with friends and family members who like to share what they order at restaurants. "You've got to try this!" they exclaim. "Hey, let me taste a bite of that," they request, fork already poised in midair. I would like to think that if Jesus were going out to dinner with me tonight, He would definitely want to share an appetizer and split a main course. Sharing is fun; however, I believe that the food Jesus ate and wants to share with us is different than we may think.

I like to imagine Jesus eating. He came to earth, fully God and fully man, which means he fully got hungry. But fish and cheese and fruits and bread weren't the things that ultimately fed Him. What enabled and empowered Jesus to keep going each day was doing the will of His Father and finishing the work God had sent Him to do.

All of food's tasty nutrients, all the energy it provides, and all the pleasure it brings pale in comparison to the satisfaction of doing God's will. That is why doing the Father's will fueled the Son.

But what exactly was the will of God that so beautifully motivated and sustained our Savior? John 6:40 tells us, "This is the will of My Father, that everyone who beholds the Son and believes in Him will have eternal life, and I Myself will raise him up on the last day" (NASB). It was God's will for Jesus to die in our place, offering us freedom in the form of forgiveness, thus securing our eternal redemption. That mission kept Jesus moving onward and upward. Like real food that gives energy to the body, our need for salvation energized our Savior. Our right to stand by His side before the Father was the driving motivation for all He did. It kept Him going.

Like real food that gives energy to the body, our need for salvation energized our Savior.

More than anything else, it is God's will that we spend our forever life with Him. His love for us is so radical that He sent His own Son to chase us down in our addictions, our compulsions, our sin, and our shame and bring us into a right relationship with Himself. The Father's will sustained the Son to carry the cross all the way up Calvary's hill. Christ was powered by the will of God! And we need to be too.

As you get more hungry for Christ, you may find yourself getting hungrier for what He hungered for. As you get to know His heart for the world, your heart for the world will be transformed to look more like His, and you will be inspired to share Him with others. Ultimately, what fueled Him will fuel you. The salvation of those you know and love and interact with each day will become a blessed burden in your belly. Like Christ, you will hunger for the salvation of the world and of your family and friends. It will become your passion, just as it was His.

We're told in Romans 8:29 that Jesus was the firstborn among us, and now it's our job to follow in His footsteps—letting the Father's purpose for Jesus's life transform our life's purpose. Isn't this what He charged us to do in the Great Commission? Before our resurrected Savior returned to the Father's side, He told His disciples—and us—to continue sharing the good news with others. He passed the baton, or passed the plate, as the case may be. It is our job now to share the news that He came to seek and to save. Let's get hungry for the salvation of the world and let that be the motivating factor in our lives today.

My oldest son is currently reading the Left Behind series for teens. He's absolutely on fire for the first time in his young life, inspired by fictional characters who are passionately sharing Christ's salvation with those who are perishing. There's an urgency to the story that most of us don't sense in our everyday lives. If we're honest, our urgency has more to do with what we will eat next and who we will eat it with and what we will wear and maybe even how we will snap a picture of it and post it to Instagram. We're motivated by what we buy and what fun activity next awaits us. We are a hungry people.

I've encouraged you before to exchange your all-consuming hunger for sweets with a new hunger: a holy hunger. Let the salvation of those who are lost fuel you. During this fast, as you begin to hunger and thirst for Christ, also let yourself hunger and thirst for opportunities to share Him with others. Offer up the food you thought you needed to eat in order to survive. Share, instead, the only thing that any of us need to truly live eternally: Christ's eternal salvation.

Let the salvation of those who are lost fuel you.

Let the will of the Father and the purpose of the Son become your food and your purpose, energizing and sustaining you through these fasting days.

The mere thought of spending forever with you sustained Jesus as He walked in sandaled feet, healing lepers and giving blind men back their sight. His love for you, dear friend, kept Him moving forward. Accept that today, if you haven't already, and let the salvation of others become your food as well.

Dear God, thank You for saving me. Help me to keep my eyes set on You as I walk out my salvation each day, looking for others to share You with. In Jesus's generous, life-giving name, Amen.

day 10

HIS PRESENCE,
OUR PRESENT

And when you fast, do not look gloomy like the hypocrites,
for they disfigure their faces that their fasting may be seen by
others. Truly, I say to you, they have received their reward. But
when you fast, anoint your head and wash your face, that your
fasting may not be seen by others but by your Father who is
in secret. And your Father who sees in secret will reward you.

Matthew 6:16–18

NUMEROUS BOOKS ABOUT FASTING smack of a pros-
perity gospel, promising that God rains down riches on our lives
when we practice this spiritual discipline. While I agree that
fasting ushers us into a life of great blessing, the more I fast,
the more I change my mind about what the blessing truly is.

Each year as I go through this fast I get quiet and, in the
quiet, the Lord brings to mind a fresh awareness of His love.
It is intimate and wonderful, and there is no greater wealth I
desire more on earth or in heaven. The same is true when I pray
and the same is true when I give. In Matthew 6, Jesus tells us

that giving and praying and fasting are *all* to be done privately rather than publicly and that a reward awaits us when we do. Like a cord of three strands carefully woven together, we are to pray and fast and give in secret. In my own life I have found that these three spiritual disciplines go hand in hand and so does the reward. They are intimately connected with one another and with God Himself.

While we tend to think that our reward for giving is that we will receive, that our reward for serving will be that we are well taken care of, and that our reward for praying will be in the form of answered prayers, I suggest, instead, that God Himself is our reward. The presence of God is our present-reward when we join Him in giving and caring for others; the nearness of God is our near-reward when we join Him in prayer; and as we empty ourselves through fasting, we experience the reward of His fullness. This intimate partnership of knowing Him and being known by Him becomes the reward much more than any earthly treasures or pleasures ever could.

> *The presence of God is our present-reward when we join Him in giving and caring for others; the nearness of God is our near-reward when we join Him in prayer; and as we empty ourselves through fasting, we experience the reward of His fullness.*

The passage I claim and cling to as my life-verse is Psalm 73:25–26, 28: "Whom have I in heaven but you? And there is nothing on earth I desire besides you. My flesh and my heart may fail, but God is the strength of my heart and my portion forever. . . . For me it is good to be near God."

Fasting brings me near God. Praying brings me near God. Giving brings me near God. When we slow down and get down on our knees, He proves Himself faithful and answers our prayers. When we join Him in sacrificial giving, we share in His work in the world and experience His heart for others. As we talk life through with Him each day, as we would a friend, His friendship is our greatest good.

God has made it clear that when we fast—or give or pray—we're not to do it in order to be seen by others. Quite the contrary. In fact, if that is our motive, our reward is forfeited. We can't keep our eyes and our hearts fixed on Him and others at the same time. Intimacy with Him, not with this world, is our goal. **We're not looking for other people's attention as we fast and give and pray; we're after God's attention and affection. That's our reward.**

I am also desperately aware of my need for Jesus when I fast, whether it's for one day or a string of days. Going without food makes me weak, and my weakness allows me to experience His strength, which is another form of reward. When I fast and pray, He proves Himself able to exceed every need that I have. His obvious nearness astounds me. His availability blows my mind. He really is present; He really is near. And there's nothing better.

The truth of this overwhelms my heart each time I fast and pray. When I am not fasting, I tend to lose sight of Him because I am running, running, running. But when I fast, I slow down and get down, low to the ground. Fasting brings me to the feet of my Savior, humble and aware of my need. Fasting reminds me that He is my Savior still, my ever-present, saving Savior.

When we are truly aware of how desperately we need Him, we have nothing to boast about. In fact, when we are fasting, boasting about it is unthinkable because true fasting only makes us aware of our need for salvation. We lack the ability to do this life without Christ at the helm. That's what we're boasting about now, one quarter of the way through this forty-day fast. It doesn't make sense to boast about how holy we are, when only Christ is our holiness. We see this most of all when we fast. That radical realization is just one more part of the precious reward.

The reward for giving and praying and fasting is found in the giving and praying and fasting. Because fasting and praying and giving allow us to experience more of Him. And He is everything. Our reward is the

The reward for giving and praying and fasting is found in the giving and praying and fasting.

intimacy forged in prayerful conversation with the One who stitched us and knows us and sits enthroned within us and over us.

As we fast from food and feast on Him, He fills the empty places in our hearts and lives with Himself. Even now, **as we go without, He goes within.**

I used to think that when Scripture talked about our rewards, it was speaking only about eternal treasures. Matthew 6:19–21 clearly tells us that there's a mighty treasure trove of blessing awaiting us in heaven: "Do not lay up for yourselves treasures on earth, where moth and rust destroy and where thieves break in and steal, but lay up for yourselves treasures in heaven, where neither moth nor rust destroys and where thieves do not break in and steal. For where your treasure is, there your heart will be also." However, now that I've been in His company on this side of glory for nearly half a century, I know that a great portion of our reward is our relationship with Him, here and now.

When we give and when we pray and when we fast, He intimately communicates with us His astounding grace, His abounding love, and His abundant goodness. He comes near to us and speaks to us clearly, as with a friend.

Are you looking for a reward as you fast and pray? **His presence is our present. His nearness, our reward.**

Dear Lord, thank You for giving me such clear directives on how to know You and experience the riches of Your presence in this present life. While I believe that You are storing up for me a heap of blessings in Your heavenly kingdom, I thank You for the gift of You, intimately near, in my life today. You are my ultimate reward! You are my gift! You are my everything. In Jesus's name, Amen.

day 11

SHINE!

You are the light of the world. A city set on a hill cannot be hidden. Nor do people light a lamp and put it under a basket, but on a stand, and it gives light to all in the house. In the same way, let your light shine before others, so that they may see your good works and give glory to your Father who is in heaven.

Matthew 5:14–16

WHETHER YOU'RE A MAN OR A WOMAN, old or young, short or tall, single or married, with children or without, you have one overarching call on your life, and that is to shine. You are called to let your light shine for Christ, wherever you are and whatever you're doing.

While that command feels nearly impossible at times, the reality is that Jesus came to show us how to be a light in the darkness. He left the glory of the kingdom of light and came to earth to live in our midst, leaving a light-drenched path for us to follow. As He walked this earth, serving and sacrificing and loving others, He referred to Himself as the Light of the World, then He passed the torch to His followers when He said, "You are the light of the world" (Matt. 5:14).

The problem is that the light in most of us has dwindled over time.

Sure, there have been seasons when we've shined unhindered, expressive, generous, bright, and bold. Others have been drawn to us at those times because we were open and welcoming and full of hope. People are drawn to light-bright individuals like a moth to a window in the black of night.

You know it's true, perhaps, but maybe it hasn't been true for you . . . recently. Somehow, during a string of long days or a season of loneliness and disappointments, your light has flickered and grown dim and maybe it's all but dead now. You feel it; you know it. Nothing in you shines bright these days. You harp on your loved ones, count the minutes until you can go to bed, retreat into social media, and hide in the pantry. When you're with people, you spend your time complaining rather than rejoicing, spreading darkness rather than shining light.

Where did your joy-light go? How did it get switched off? There are too many reasons to count and too many shadows darkening your life and snuffing out your testimony: the worries of this world, the challenges of marriage and child rearing, financial stresses, broken hearts, broken dreams, dashed expectations, and an unhealthy lifestyle full of unhealthy habits. All these things can overwhelm you, zap your energy, and throw your emotions out of balance, hiding the light of Christ within you.

I'm reminded of a song I used to sing in Sunday school that went like this, "This little light of mine, I'm going to let it shine. This little light of mine, I'm going to let it shine, let it shine, let it shine, let it shine. Hide it under a bushel? No! I'm going to let it shine. Hide it under a bushel? No! I'm going to let it shine, let it shine, let it shine, let it shine."

While I am not here to address all the "bushels" that may be hiding your light, I do want to invite you to invite Jesus, the Light of the World, back into the dreary corners and dark recesses of your heart today. He is the Light and He promises that when you walk with Him, you'll not walk another step in darkness.

> Again Jesus spoke to them, saying, "I am the light of the world. Whoever follows me will not walk in darkness, but will have the light of life." (John 8:12)

Have you been struggling in the dark? Maybe your dearest friend has died, your marriage has ended, your health is failing, or your inner dialogue is one long monologue of self-loathing. Sin and soul-sadness thrive in the dark. But God promises that if you fetter yourself to Him and walk by His side, you will walk in His life-light. And like Moses, whose face shone with the brightness of God after he stood face-to-face in His presence for forty days (Exod. 34:35), you will start to shine again. That's what these forty days are for.

He is the Light and He promises that when you walk with Him, you'll not walk another step in darkness.

Friends, in this life we will encounter many dark trials, but we can be of good cheer—and cheer is a lot like shining—for our Savior has overcome the world and is overcoming still. His love and overcoming goodness radiates off our faces as we abide in Him. So don't go moping about as you fast, complaining about your withdrawal symptoms and all the sacrifices you're making so that God draws near. Splash some water on your face and shine. Shine amongst your family members during these forty days. Your spouse and children and neighbors and coworkers should have to shield their eyes because you're suddenly so radiant and bright. You're not only reflecting His light but it is also coming from within you now! You've got light down in your core because you're plugged into the light source.

> Let your light shine before others, so that they may see your good works and give glory to your Father who is in heaven. (Matt. 5:16)

Are you able to let your light shine before others today? If not, I encourage you to run back into the presence of the Light of the World. If you have been complaining this past week, be quiet today. Take a shower and go for a walk and speak grateful blessings over your life and the lives of those around you. Look for new ways to love and serve. If your children and your spouse have been demanding and you've responded to them with nasty words and expressions, ask the Lord to shine His love in you and through you. Let the Holy Spirit shine in your home. If you are lonely, go to the One who can fill each hollow hurt with His holy healing.

In this life we will encounter many dark trials, but we can be of good cheer . . . for our Savior has overcome the world and is overcoming still.

And if you grumble every time you walk into the breakroom at work and see a plate of cookies, turn around and take your break somewhere else. When you're able, walk back in there and shine without complaining.

You are the light of the world—so shine.

Dear Light of the World, shine in me and shine through me today as I commit to walking with You. Amen!

day 12

FOOD TRIGGERS

Search me, O God, and know my heart!
Try me and know my thoughts!
And see if there be any grievous way in me,
and lead me in the way everlasting!
Psalm 139:23–24

IN 2016, my friend Amber Lia and I were ministering online
to overwhelmed moms who were struggling with anger. In our
private Facebook group Amber and I shared biblical, practical parenting advice and told stories of our own challenges
with our kids. One day we asked this simple question: "What
are your triggers?" There was no need to define what a trigger
was; these moms knew. Within an hour, hundreds of women
responded: "When my kids talk back." "When they whine."
"Sibling rivalry!" "Why can't they get their shoes on and get
in the car?" "Naptime." "Bedtime." "Dinnertime." "My messy
house." "My messy life."

Amber and I didn't try to teach those moms how to train their
kids to behave better so that they wouldn't get angry. Instead
we focused on our need to submit our triggered hearts to the

gentle lordship of Jesus Christ—only then can our triggers lose their tight hold on our hearts. After months of addressing each trigger one at a time, Amber and I published a book, which we aptly titled *Triggers: Exchanging Parents' Angry Reactions for Gentle Biblical Responses.* I share this now to convey that I understand what it means to be triggered—triggered internally by our emotions and triggered externally by our circumstances.

Most of us have food triggers as well. **When our triggers are out of control, so is our eating.** As a matter of fact, the National Institute for Mental Health has confirmed that binge eating is the most common eating disorder in America today.[1] Even if we don't consider ourselves clinical cases, I bet we can each put a finger on a trigger or two that sets us off and causes us to eat compulsively or emotionally.

Perhaps your food trigger is your sensitive feelings, and you use food to comfort yourself each time you feel wronged or angry. Or maybe your trigger is a desperate desire to feel loved or the memory of a past hurt. Food triggers abound but we need wisdom to know which ones have mastery over us.

I often pray Psalm 139 when asking the Lord to give me spiritual vision to pinpoint my own food triggers. I ask Him to search me, acknowl-edging that He knows me better than I know myself. He made me and I am His—hurts, habits, and all. He isn't angry with me but loves me unconditionally. He wants to heal me from unhealthy eating, living, and thinking, so I invite Him to reveal anything that's harmful or offensive in me that He wants to make right. Humbly I ask Him to lead me in the everlasting way.

He made me and I am His—hurts, habits, and all.

Have you asked Jesus to reveal to you why it is that you overindulge on sugar? He can show you what your triggers are. Maybe He'll give you eyes to see that when your children melt down at 3:00 p.m. and you're tempted to melt down too, you turn to chocolate chips rather than to Him. You open the refrigerator rather than opening the Word. Or perhaps He'll show you that when your spouse isn't showing you love and respect, you run to food to relieve the hurt. Take a moment to consider your food triggers.

While I've intentionally focused on the spiritual side of things during this fast, there is a physical side to our love for sugar as well. Physiologically, when you ingest sugar, dopamine floods your body making you feel happy and hopeful. If you struggle with sadness every day, dopamine feels like a savior. Unfortunately, the happiness quickly retreats and the mournful feelings return, spiraling you downward again. The next time you turn to food to relieve your emotional sadness, you need a larger portion to achieve the same result. After a while, the body stops releasing dopamine without the assistance of sugar (or sex or drugs or anything else you've trained your body to respond to). That is why sugar is addictive. Your body actually becomes dependent upon sugar to complete its natural function and release the feel-good chemical of dopamine. How sad.

Another physiological reason people overeat is that many foods have been synthetically engineered and genetically modified to become an addictive substance. While this might not have been the intention of engineers, it has been a direct result of modern chemical innovations. In his book *Wheat Belly*, cardiologist and author William Davis tells us that there is actually an addictive ingredient in wheat today that keeps people coming back for more. Here is how he summed it up on his blog:

> Modern wheat is an opiate. And, of course, I don't mean that wheat is an opiate in the sense that you like it so much that you

feel you are addicted. *Wheat is truly addictive.* . . . But the "high" of wheat is not like the high of heroin, morphine, or OxyContin. This opiate, while it binds to the opiate receptors of the brain, doesn't make us high. It makes us *hungry*.

This is the effect exerted by *gliadin*, the protein in wheat that was inadvertently altered by geneticists in the 1970s during efforts to increase yield. Just a few shifts in amino acids and gliadin in modern high-yield, semi-dwarf wheat became *a potent appetite stimulant.*[2]

Simply put, certain foods can make us hungrier. I'm reminded of the Lay's Potato Chips slogan that challenged, "Bet you can't eat just one!" This is what we're up against physically as we go to battle spiritually. Food, the very thing God created to satisfy our physical hunger, has been engineered to stimulate it! That's just one more reason why food triggers abound.

Food, the very thing God created to satisfy our physical hunger, has been engineered to stimulate it!

Ironically, the first group of people I invited to join me for this 40-Day Sugar Fast were actually the same overwhelmed moms in the Facebook group I wrote about earlier. They immediately recognized that their emotional triggers weren't just causing them to get angry with their kids, they were pushing them to run to food to cope with their stress. And the sugar they consumed made them even more emotionally unstable than before. Those moms knew that they needed a physical detox and a spiritual fast!

One woman who joined me for that first fast was my friend Asheritah Ciuciu. A few years later she published a book entitled *Full: Food, Jesus, and the Battle for Satisfaction.* In chapter 7 of her book, Asheritah focuses solely on food triggers. She begins,

"It's useful for us to determine what our particular triggers are, and when faced with that trigger, we can make the intentional choice of whether to go to God or go to food."[3] Pinpointing your personal food triggers is one of the most practical and helpful things you can do if you want to learn to turn to Christ when triggered. Asheritah suggests keeping a running log of the times you find yourself desperate to put something into your mouth so that you can see the patterns and identify your personal food triggers. Perhaps you'll discover that you are tempted to binge only at night once the kids are finally asleep. Or maybe your triggers appear at work when you're struggling to complete a big project. Once you identify your triggers, you won't be powerless against them. You'll be able to make a plan and choose how to cope with them in a healthy way.

As you look back over the past twelve days of your fast, consider when you were most tempted to cave. Was it out of stress or sadness? Did you feel out of control in your parenting or unattractive and unloved in your most intimate relationship? Ask the Lord to search you and know you and reveal to you when you're tempted to turn to food instead of to Him. Then take it one step further and come up with a better plan. Commit to recognizing the underlying feelings and take them to the Lord. With His help, you can also build a healthier and holier habit to combat your most triggered moments.

Dear Lord, search me and know my hungry heart today. Try me and know my triggered thoughts. See if there are any unhealthy habits in my eating and my thinking and my living, and lead me in the everlasting way. I invite You, Lord, to reveal to me why it is I run to food instead of You. Teach me that You are what I need every time I'm triggered. In Jesus's name, Amen.

day 13

WEIGHT AND WORSHIP

But seek first the kingdom of God and his righteousness, and
all these things will be added to you.

Matthew 6:33

THERE'S NOTHING WRONG with wanting to lose the
extra weight you may be carrying around, whether the extra
load comes from literal pounds or from pounds of pain. However, **for deep and lasting physical and emotional transformation to occur, you first need deep and lasting spiritual
transformation.** Matthew 6:33 makes it clear: **When you turn
your eyes, first and foremost, on God, everything else will fall
into its rightful place.** Conversely, when you look to the scale
first, it's nearly impossible to see past it to the soul.

When you're tempted to obsess about your weight, ask yourself this: Which will last forever—my spirit or my body? Of
course, you know that your body will wear out and your flesh
and bones will pass away. But have you considered the never-
ending expansiveness of your soul? **Though God's Spirit takes
up residency within you when you put your faith in Jesus,
your skin isn't His eternal dwelling place—nor is it yours.
It's your spirit that dwells with Him.**

Eventually we will leave our bodies and receive glorified bodies. Philippians 3:21 promises: "He will take our weak mortal bodies and change them into glorious bodies like his own, using the same power with which he will bring everything under his control" (NLT). When we get to heaven, we will see God face-to-face—our new forever face to His eternal face. But for now, He is deep within us, looking at us spirit-to-spirit. He is gazing, eyes fixed, at the eternal spirit within us, so we must turn our attention to what He's most passionate about—our spirit's rightness. One million years from now our spirits will still be with His Spirit. Oh, the thought of it!

Those of us who have walked through these forty days before have discovered that when we seek Him first—when we fast from sugar in order to feast on Him—the pounds often start falling off. When we think about the fullness of Christ in us, we stop thinking so much about filling ourselves with food. When we long for the One who truly satisfies, we tend to stop turning to momentary fillers.

Do you see where I'm going with this? The natural man turns his attention to his natural body first: his diet, his exercise, his New Year's resolution. The natural woman steps onto the scale and counts her steps. But weigh this concept carefully. What if we stop counting our steps and start walking in step with God instead? What if we run to Him before we take a run around the block?

Let me be clear. I am not saying you should forget about your physical well-being. Whether your body is oversized or under-nourished is important, and you need to take good care of it. You need cardiovascular exercise for heart health and strength training for muscle health. You need to drink plenty of water too for healthy, hydrated cells and muscles. These are all good things to do. But the starting point for your whole health does not begin with *whole foods* but with *holiness*.

Christ didn't die for your hips or your bust or your belly. He died so that your spirit would remain with Him now and forever. While your body will fail, your spirit will never wear out from age or gravity. That's why you need to spend more time considering the rightness of your spirit and the righteousness of God rather than how right or wrong you think your body is. Do you need more exercise? Perhaps. But running to Jesus has to be your number one form of cardio.

Your eternal spirit is the Holy Spirit's chief concern.

It's easy to obsess over our personal appearance, because we live in a culture obsessed with appearance. However, 1 Samuel 16:7 reminds us, "The LORD does not look at the things people look at. People look at the outward appearance, but the LORD looks at the heart" (NIV).

In order to keep our spiritual health in focus, we have to keep the Spirit in focus. We must seek Him before all else. Though the unseen Spirit of God seems elusive, He is the fullness of God in our daily lives. We need a steady diet of seeking Him and finding Him at the forefront of all we do each day. In Jeremiah 29:13, God promises us, "You will seek me and find me when you seek me with all your heart." Deuteronomy 4:29 tells us, "But if from there you seek the LORD your God, you will find him if you seek him with all your heart and with all your soul" (NIV). We're given even more assurance of His promises in 2 Chronicles 15:4, "But when they in their trouble did turn unto the LORD God of Israel, and sought him, he was found of them" (KJV).

Over and over again throughout the Scriptures God tells us that when we turn to Him, we will find Him. But the miracle gets even more miraculous! When we give the Spirit of God access to our spiritual lives, He lovingly addresses the present reality of our physical and emotional lives too. He doesn't say, "Good! You've got heaven now, that's enough"; instead, He says, "In light of our eternity together, let's deal with this present life together."

You're living two lives now: a temporary existence bound up in the flesh and an everlasting life bound up in the spirit. Much of this Christian life is learning how those two lives flow together. I have personally found that when I focus on that which is fleeting, I lose sight of that which will last. However, when my eyes are fixed on my eternal life, I have a deep sense that the Lord cares deeply about my present life too.

When you seek Him first, you can trust Him with the rest. When you seek the eternal God, you can trust Him with even the temporary struggles. Pounds and pain melt away in a red-hot relationship with the eternal Son. Seek Him spiritually, and you will see what He can do in you physically.

When our lives begin to change from the inside out, our eating habits will change from the outside in. That's why this book doesn't focus on what we can eat each day. We're seeking Him first and foremost. These daily readings are the soul food we need. The problems of this world—whether to do with weight, relationships, finances, popularity, or emotional and physical health—will pass away, but God's righteousness stretches from the past to the present and points us toward forever. Worship His righteousness today.

> *When our lives begin to change from the inside out, our eating habits will change from the outside in.*

Seek Him and find Him! Get into His righteousness and His righteousness will get into you, satisfying as nothing else can.

Dear Lord, help me take this Scripture from Matthew 6:33 and hide it in my heart and believe it when I start to chase after all the other things first: "Seek first the kingdom of God and his righteousness, and all these things will be added to you." I'm trusting You with all things as I learn to seek You first. Because of Your Son and in His name, Amen.

day 14

WHAT ELSE ARE YOU CRAVING?

For you created my inmost being;
you knit me together in my mother's womb.

Psalm 139:13 NIV

HALFWAY THROUGH my last forty-day fast, I mindlessly opened up one of my children's apps on my phone and started playing a game. It wasn't a game I'd played before, but I was bored and it caught my eye as I waited for a load of laundry to finish tumbling in the dryer. Two hours later, I looked at the clock and saw that it was time to pick my sons up from school. I hadn't finished doing the laundry or started preparing for dinner, so I was agitated and short-tempered with the boys when I brought them home from school. Their banter and efforts to get my attention only annoyed me, and I finally retreated into the bathroom where I played yet another round of my new game!

True, I hadn't run to food to distract me—after all, I was fasting from sugar!—but I also had not turned to the Lord. I **had crammed something new into the empty places sugar**

left behind. I had consumed a new distraction and numbed my annoyance with a new medicine.

Have you found yourself doing the same? Exchanging one false filler for another? You are now two weeks into your fast; perhaps some of the other addictions that have been simmering on the back burner of your life are moving to the forefront. Or maybe you've found yourself turning to something entirely new. Either way, I want to encourage you to look beyond your sugar addiction so that you can see what else you might be running to.

Picture sugar as the doorway through which you invite the Holy Spirit to come into the private, innermost places of your life. Imagine Him now, deep within your heart, looking around and taking inventory. See Him smiling as He says, "Thanks for the sugar, but I want it all." What started as a sugar fast has the potential to be so much more. I'm praying that God will give you the eyes to see other hidden idols in your life in the days ahead. Layer after layer, as you seek God in His Word, allow Him to convict you of other stuff you may be turning to.

Scottish minister Andrew Bonar said, "Fasting is abstaining from anything that hinders prayer."[1] Not just food. *Anything.* As a matter of fact, Bonar often fasted from reading in order to spend more time with the Lord. *Reading!* His example ought to challenge us to consider what else might be hindering our intimate friendship with the Lord. If we want to experience His sustaining hand in our lives, it may be a good idea to take a season to set aside anything that might be in *our* hands. I like to say it this way: We abstain so that He might sustain. This isn't just about food. We don't just run to the pantry—we run to online games, we run to romance novels, and we run to Starbucks too.

We abstain so that He might sustain.

When we regularly run to anything or anyone else other than Christ to meet our deepest needs, we find only a temporary solution. Christ, however, is eternal. He satisfies us as nothing else can because He is intimately acquainted with each and every part of our souls. After all, He created our innermost beings. Psalm 139:13 tells us clearly, "For you created my inmost being; you knit me together in my mother's womb" (NIV). He made us and He knows us, and He knows what will truly satisfy and fill us.

> Now on the last day, the great day of the feast, Jesus stood and cried out, saying, "If anyone is thirsty, let him come to Me and drink. He who believes in Me, as the Scripture said, 'From his innermost being will flow rivers of living water.'" (John 7:37–38 NASB)

If we want our innermost places filled to overflowing, we've got to turn to God instead of food or other false fillers. In John chapter 7, *innermost being* has been translated from the Greek word *koilia*, which is often used to describe one's belly. However, it not only represents the physical cavity of the stomach but also the emotional seat, which in English we consider our heart.[2] In the above passage, Jesus describes a spiritual emptiness in the heart of humankind, not a physical hunger in one's belly. He understands it because He made us. **The One who made our core is the only One able to fill it.**

Today, as you move deeper into fasting, ask yourself: "Is there anything else that I'm running to? Is there anything else that I need to lay down? Am I turning to anything or anyone else to fill the God hole within me?"

Physicist and theologian Blaise Pascal wrote:

> What is it, then, that this desire and this inability proclaim to us, but that there was once in man a true happiness of which

there now remain to him only the mark and empty trace, which he in vain tries to fill from all his surroundings, seeking from things absent the help he does not obtain in things present? But these are all inadequate, because the infinite abyss can only be filled by an infinite and immutable object, that is to say, only by God Himself.[3]

These words from Pascal inspired the American evangelist Bill Bright to pen this famous statement: "There is a God-shaped vacuum in the heart of every man which cannot be filled by any created thing, but only by God the Creator, made known through Jesus Christ."[4] If this is true, and I believe that it is, then we should be more excited about the fruits of this fast than words can express. God is eager to rush into all the empty places we long to fill. God has the power to turn our hollow places into a hallowed place.

God has the power to turn our hollow places into a hallowed place.

First we must recognize that the Creator made us to crave Him. So often we misunderstand the hunger in our hearts, the grumbling deep inside us, and we turn to the wrong stuff. Lysa TerKeurst, author of *Made to Crave*, said it this way, "God made us to crave—to desire eagerly, want greatly, and long for Him. But Satan wants to do everything possible to replace our craving for God with something else."[5]

Let's not underestimate the devil as we fast and pray in the weeks ahead. You might have picked this book up simply to help you as you detox your body. I urge you to not only offer God the food you consume but also to offer Him everything you turn to instead of Him. Perhaps you turn to those you "like" online rather than the One who loves you to the cross and back. Perhaps you run to the store when you could be storing up treasures in heaven. What do you turn to for satisfaction each time your innermost being cries out for Jesus? Are you restless to fill the void? What you live to fill, Christ died to fill! The satisfied life is yours for the taking if you want it.

What started as a sugar fast can be so much more. What else do you need to surrender for the remainder of this fast?

Dear Lord, I know that sugar isn't the only thing I turn to when I could turn to You. Prick my heart with conviction in the days ahead as I consider what else it is that I'm running to instead of You! You made me to crave You, but I need Your help to set all my other cravings on the altar first. Humbly, Holy Spirit, I'm asking for Your help. Amen.

day 15

DIVISIVE DEVICES

My people have committed two sins:
They have forsaken me,
   the spring of living water,
and have dug their own cisterns,
   broken cisterns that cannot hold water.

Jeremiah 2:13 NIV

THERE WAS A TIME when I slept with my thin, brown Bible under my pillow. It was during one of the hardest seasons of my life—when loneliness threatened to undo me. I would go to sleep with my head literally resting upon my Bible and my heart resting there too. It was symbolic, perhaps, but all I knew was that I needed it close.

In the morning, when the sun rose, I'd reach my hand under my pillow before wiping the sleep from my eyes. My Bible was my daily bread because I was so hungry for love. I'd open it up and start reading where I had left off the night before. **Verse after verse, chapter after chapter, God's Word flooded into all the hurting places of my heart.**

I did this until my husband and I were happily married. That's when I moved my Bible from beneath my pillow to beside my bed. In the morning I would wake up, stretch, reach for my Bible, and then continue reading where I had last left off.

Ten years after we were married, I got my first smartphone. I plugged it in and charged it beside my bed, right beside my Bible. Since my phone held both my alarm clock and my Bible app, it was easy to pick up and open up. The trouble was, all the notifications from the night hours would immediately catch my eye. Before I knew it, instead

Verse after verse, chapter after chapter, God's Word flooded into all the hurting places of my heart.

of spending the early moments of my day with the Lord, I was spending them online with everyone but Him. I found myself eager to know what my friends had to say to me before I turned my attention to what God had to say to me. The temptation was both subtle and obvious.

Each time I host the 40-Day Sugar Fast online, I receive hundreds of letters with confessions like this: "I know that sugar is a struggle for me, but my real addiction is to my phone." My friend, author Katie M. Reid, joined me in the fast one year. She publicly confessed her own temptation to turn to social media over and over again each day, though she longed to turn with such fervor and consistency to the Lord. She pointed out the apple on the back of most of our phones, and we all saw her point. No wonder there's a bite taken out of that apple! Just as Eve was tempted away from God's best plan for her life, we feel the pull of temptation too.

Our smartphones can keep us connected to the world, but they can't keep us connected to Christ. They can keep track of our schedules, but they can't order our priorities. They can play our praise music with a single voice command, but they cannot fill our souls with praise.

Jeremiah 2:13 is the verse I'd like you to focus on today, and the verse I try to keep at the forefront of my life. "My people have committed two sins: They have forsaken me, the spring of living water, and have dug their own cisterns, broken cisterns that cannot hold water" (NIV).

His water is both cleansing and satisfying, and those who take a long, cool drink from the well of His saving grace will never thirst again.

Jesus called Himself the living water. His water is both cleansing and satisfying, and those who take a long, cool drink from the well of His saving grace will never thirst again.

You and I both know that it is easy to forsake that well of living water and dig for ourselves other wells. Other cisterns. But they are broken and can't even hold water.

> In your distress you called and I rescued you,
> I answered you out of a thundercloud;
> I tested you at the waters of Meribah.
> Hear me, my people, and I will warn you—
> if you would only listen to me, Israel!
> You shall have no foreign god among you;
> you shall not worship any god other than me.
> I am the LORD your God,
> who brought you up out of Egypt.
> Open wide your mouth and I will fill it.
> But my people would not listen to me;
> Israel would not submit to me.
> So I gave them over to their stubborn hearts
> to follow their own devices. (Ps. 81:7–12 NIV)

Oh, what a powerful passage as the Lord reminded His people of just how faithful He had been. They cried out in their distress and He answered them. Immediately He tested them and reminded them to stay close and to continue to listen. He warned them not to go looking for foreign gods because He is the God who saved them for Himself. He offered to feed them. "Open wide your mouth," He said, "and I will fill it" (v. 10). But they turned away and would not listen and would not eat from His hand nor drink from His cup. Eventually, He gave them over to their own "devices."

Do you see the similarities between the Israelites and the people so attached to their technology today? Devices—it's what we call our smartphones and tablets, our computers and iPads. Oh how divisive they can be when they become our electronic, foreign gods, dividing us from the one true God. Sugar isn't the only idol to which we turn. This fast isn't simply about cutting out sugar; it's about abstaining from anything and everything we've learned to run to time and again.

Ask the God who redeemed you to show you what devices are dividing you from Him, and consider fasting from them during the remaining weeks of your fast. Perhaps its as simple as removing all the social media apps off of your phone or charging it in the bathroom rather than on your bedside table for the next twenty-five days. Then, once your fast is over, maybe you'll set some boundaries to keep God on the throne of your life—and everything else in its rightful place.

Dear Lord, I want You to be the only thing I thirst for, because You are the only One who can ever truly satisfy. All the other fillers seem to intensify my desire for more, but You alone can fill me to overflowing! Show me where I've manufactured for myself broken cisterns that can't hold water—let alone living water. In Jesus's quenching name, Amen.

THE 40-DAY SOCIAL MEDIA FAST

If you are convicted that your phone is even more addictive than sugar, you aren't alone. Find out about the 40-Day Social Media Fast at 40daysocialmediafast.com.

day 16

COMFORT FOODS AND RETAIL THERAPY

Blessed be the God and Father of our Lord Jesus Christ, the Father of mercies and God of all comfort, who comforts us in all our affliction, so that we may be able to comfort those who are in any affliction, with the comfort with which we ourselves are comforted by God.

2 Corinthians 1:3–4

WE ARE SIXTEEN DAYS into this forty-day fast from sugar, and you may think I'm backsliding but stick with me. *There's nothing wrong with sweet treats.* Let's not forget that the promised land was flowing with honey! Dates and grapes, all full to bursting with natural sugars, hung heavy on trees and vines, with honeybees buzzing all around. Throughout the Old Testament, kings, warriors, lovers, and prophets ate honey and it revived them. What a sweet gift from God!

Honey isn't simply packed with natural sugars that provide a quick surge of energy, and it doesn't merely sweeten our tea. When applied to the skin, honey can heal wounds. When applied to the throat, it soothes pain. Few things are richer in vitamins, minerals, proteins, fatty acids, enzymes, and bioflavonoids than the sweet honey produced by the honey-making bee.

God, in His kindness, gave us honey from the comb, and He likened it to His Word because it is sweet and satisfying. It nourishes our bodies and revives us when we are in desperate need of revival. However, Proverbs 25:16 warns: "Have you found honey? Eat only what you need, that you do not have it in excess and vomit it" (NASB).

The lesson today isn't simply moderation; it's that honey isn't the promised land. It's a gift of the promise but it's not the promise in and of itself. When we think that sugar—whether natural or refined—is the promised land, we miss the promised land entirely. Likewise, when we run to food for our comfort, we miss out on the Great Comforter. "I am he who comforts you" (Isa. 51:12).

Perhaps you started fasting because of a few extra pounds, but you're recognizing that you're actually carrying around loads of pain. Maybe a parent abandoned you or your spouse betrayed you. Perhaps you were verbally, physically, or sexually abused. No matter the source of the hurt, old wounds create a lonely ache that needs a comforting touch. Some hurts leave deep, dark holes that fester, raw and aching.

Many people have learned to self-medicate their pain with food. Perhaps you run to brownies or caramels—or caramel brownies—for relief, only to find that it used to take one or two to lift you up and make you happy again, but now it takes half a pan to soothe the hurt. And even then the anesthesia doesn't last long. I know because I've done these things myself. When you turn to food for pain management, the pain is not healed but only masked for a time.

I also know plenty of people who use retail therapy as a way to make themselves feel better. But believe it or not, Target

COMFORT FOODS AND RETAIL THERAPY **99**

isn't the promised land either (gasp). If you run to the store when you are feeling bored or lonely, only to come out with a bag of clothes or new cosmetics, you might feel a temporary high, but it won't last. A full cart never makes a heart full. Shopping may help you feel better for the afternoon, but your credit card statements will last longer than the effects of your retail therapy. Before you know it, you will be sad or unhappy or bored again, and your wallet can't cover the cost of the ongoing pain. When you try to soothe the hurt with purchases, new pain arises. Even if you're not going into debt, you can't afford to keep purchasing this way because it's getting in the way of what you need most spiritually.

Here's the thing: Comfort food and retail therapy can never bring us anything more than temporary relief. It is only when we run to an eternal God that we find lasting comfort. Sweets and new purchases may be able to revive our hearts for the moment but only He can revive us internally and eternally. We need a true revival more than an ephemeral food or shopping high. We need the promised land of God in our lives, not just the sweet treats He's included in the bounty.

Comfort food and retail therapy can never bring us anything more than temporary relief.

Jesus came to earth to chase us down in our pain and to heal us of our diseases. He walked with the disciples and talked with them too. He went to the cross and died for all our sins. He rose again, overcoming the tyranny of sin and sadness in every desperate life. During Jesus's final days on earth, He stayed with the disciples and ministered to them. When He left to return to the Father, He gave them His Spirit with these words: "And I will pray the Father, and he shall give you another Comforter, that he may abide with you for ever" (John 14:16 KJV).

If you are sad today and have been sad for a long time, open your Bible and ingest the sweetness of John 14, which begins, "Do not let your hearts be troubled" (NIV). When you learn to run to the Comforter, He will fill you with His comfort. You will be filled to overflowing when you take your hungry-for-comfort heart to Him! Eventually, you will be so full of comfort that He will make you an ambassador of His

His comfort won't simply fill you, it will overflow from you and fill others who are sad as well.

comfort. You won't be able to stop yourself from sharing His goodness with others. His comfort won't simply fill you, it will overflow from you and fill others who are sad as well. When God comforts you, He makes you a comforter; His healing makes you a healer; and His saving makes you a walking, talking testimonial to His saving grace. **When you encounter the promised land of life in Christ, healed and whole, you become ambassadors of His promises.**

Shopping doesn't satisfy. Brownies don't either. Only the great Comforter does. Commit, my friends, to staying close to the Spirit of all comfort each day of this fast, for your benefit and the benefit of others.

Dear Lord, Your kindness to me is beyond my understanding. You've filled the land with sweet and satisfying things. And yet, You are the sweetest and most satisfying of all. Teach my heart to long for You and come to You. Train my legs to run to You! For You are my promised land, my Comforter, my Healer, my Savior God. Amen.

day 17

BE QUIET AND BE TRANSFORMED

Don't shoot off your mouth or speak before you think. Don't be too quick to tell God what you think he wants to hear. God's in charge, not you—the less you speak, the better.

Ecclesiastes 5:2 MSG

EUGENE PETERSON, author of the poetic Message adaptation of the Bible, passed away in 2018. He brought the antiquated language of God's Word to life for many of us. In Matthew 17 he added descriptive details to the story of Jesus's transfiguration in front of His close friends. The idea of Christ's transformation captured my imagination the first time that I read these words: "His appearance changed from the inside out, right before their eyes. Sunlight poured from his face. His clothes were filled with light" (Matt. 17:2 MSG). **Christ's fully-God persona burned through the thin veil of flesh that made Him fully man.**

Can you imagine what it must have been like for Peterson to first describe our Savior's bright and blinding presence upon the mountaintop with His disciples, and then to actually be the disciple looking into Jesus's transfigured face? Brilliant and blinding and beautiful!

One day you will see Jesus face-to-face as well. If you have put your faith in the Son, you will stand before Him in His kingdom of light. Jesus, who first made the earth then walked upon it, will walk right up to you. His light will shine upon you. In His bright transfigured presence, you will be transfigured too.

We're told that Jesus is the lamp of heaven, the source who lights our eternal dwelling home. "The city does not need the sun or the moon to shine on it, for the glory of God gives it light, and the Lamb is its lamp" (Rev. 21:23 NIV). That's the light that blazed through our Savior from the inside out on the mount of transfiguration. That same light has the power to transfigure us! The real miracle is that we don't have to wait to encounter Him in heaven either. The same God who was transformed on earth is willing and able to transform us on earth.

The subtitle of this book, *Where Physical Detox Meets Spiritual Transformation*, is a promise. Transformation through Christ is so much more than pressing a physical restart button. **When you stop running to food and start running to the transfigured Savior, He transforms not only your figure but your heart as well!** But food isn't the only thing that stops us from running to Him. Sometimes we're so busy running our mouths that we miss out on what He's saying and what He's doing.

Consider Peter's response to seeing Jesus talking with Elijah and Moses.

> Jesus took Peter and the brothers, James and John, and led them up a high mountain. His appearance changed from the inside out, right before their eyes. Sunlight poured from his face. His clothes were filled with light. Then they realized that Moses and Elijah were also there in deep conversation with him.

Peter broke in, "Master, this is a great moment! What would you think if I built three memorials here on the mountain—one for you, one for Moses, one for Elijah?"

While he was going on like this, babbling, a light-radiant cloud enveloped them, and sounding from deep in the cloud a voice: "This is my Son, marked by my love, focus of my delight. Listen to him." (Matt. 17:1–5 MSG)

While I'd like to think that my first response to the glory pouring from Jesus's face would be to fall prostrate, perhaps I'd do what Peter did instead. He leaped into action—interrupting Jesus and making plans to build memorials. He continued babbling until God told him to be quiet. **The Father told Peter to stop speaking and listen to His Son.**

All my talking and all my planning can get in the way of hearing God's good plan for me.

Today I'm thinking about my own need to pipe down and listen. My desire to be physically transformed can get in the way of me quietly and humbly worshiping the One who was transformed and has the power to transform me! All my plans to get to the gym and get on the scale and stay on a diet (and all my meal plans too) pale in comparison to the brilliant transforming power of God at work in my life. All my talking and all my planning can get in the way of hearing God's good plan for me.

As you fast, let me encourage you to stop talking and start listening. **Stop running your mouth and start running to Him with ears to hear.** Author Bob Sorge wrote these challenging words in his book *The Secrets of the Secret Place*: "Hearing God's voice has become the singular quest of my heart, the sole pursuit that alone satisfies the great longings of my heart."[1] You have committed to intentionally lay down for forty days that which cannot satisfy in order to experience the only One who can. His voice satisfies. Hearing Him and doing what He says is the secret that can be found only in the quiet of a listening heart.

Do you need to fast from talking for the next few weeks? I don't mean twenty-four hours a day, but maybe one holy hour each morning in order to hear the Lord whispering to your spirit. Sorge goes on to say, "I strongly advocate for a prayer life that is comprised mostly of silence. It's a great delight to talk to God, but it's even more thrilling when He talks to us. I've discovered that He has more important things to say than I do. Things don't change when I talk to God; things change when God talks to me. When I talk, nothing happens; when God talks, the universe comes into existence."[2]

Be quiet. Be listening. Be transformed.

Over the course of the next twenty-three days, spend more time quietly ingesting His transforming Word than you spend speaking words. Spend more time listening to Him than you spend talking. Hear the Father say, "This is my Son, marked by my love, focus of my delight. Listen to him" (MSG). Be quiet. Be listening. Be transformed.

Dear Lord, You are magnificent. You are beautiful and Your Words transform all who listen and receive. I want to hear from You more than I want to talk to You about my plan each day of this fast. Teach me to quiet down so that I might be satisfied by Your voice. I can only imagine what it will be like to stand transformed before Your light-drenched countenance in Your eternal kingdom of light! Until that day, Lord, slowly but surely transform me into Your likeness. I'll be quietly trusting You with the process. In Jesus's name, Amen.

day 18

STUMBLING BLOCKS AND DYNAMITE

If your right eye causes you to stumble, gouge it out and throw it away. It is better for you to lose one part of your body than for your whole body to be thrown into hell. And if your right hand causes you to stumble, cut it off and throw it away. It is better for you to lose one part of your body than for your whole body to go into hell.

Matthew 5:29–30 NIV

YOU ARE NEARLY HALFWAY through your fast. Perhaps the nasty withdrawal migraines you were experiencing are gone and have been replaced with increased energy and more stable emotions. I hope so. However, I don't want you to rest on the laurels of what you've received so far. You may have lost a few pounds, but there's so much more to be gained! Gaining more often requires losing more, and now I'm not talking about pounds at all. If there are other things in your life standing between you and God, today's the day to cast them down.

In Matthew 5:30, Jesus says, "If your right hand causes you to stumble, cut it off and throw it away. It is better for you to lose one part of your body than for your whole body to go into hell" (NIV). One of the problems with familiar Bible passages like this one is that you can read them quickly and move on unchanged. However, the subtitle of this book promises spiritual transformation, which means change has to occur. If there is anything in your life that is causing you to stumble in your journey to be with God and like God, today is the day you stop tripping over it. You've given Him your sugar, and that's no small thing; you've considered your smartphone and other devices; you've surrendered your credit card and your constant go-go-going; but perhaps there is something else that's standing in the way and keeping you from feasting on Him.

Not all stumbling blocks are idols. Some things simply trip us up because we like them a little too much and our attention is pulled off course.

Not all stumbling blocks are idols. Some things simply trip us up because we like them a little too much and our attention is pulled off course. With a little conviction, however, we're back on track with healthy boundaries again. While not everything that causes us to stumble is an idol, idols can bring us down faster than anything else.

Years ago I learned to recognize an idol in my life by answering this one simple question: Would taking away _____ devastate me? Would having to give up Instagram wreck my life? Would foregoing dessert make me an emotional basket case? Would laying down my hobby for a season feel like laying down my life forever? Could I give up hosting annual family gatherings during the holidays and let my sister-in-law do it? Could I say no to a nightly glass or two of wine without panic attacks?

Could I leave my volunteer position at the church or the humane society or my child's school without losing my sense of identity? If the answer is "No, I could not do that without extreme emotional stress," then I know that I have discovered an idol—a massive blockade standing between me and God.

Consider your hobbies, the things you spend your time and money doing. While there is nothing inherently wrong with having a hobby, when your passions and pleasures become preeminent, taking up your first priority spot, you've got it backward. And walking backward is a lot like stumbling blindly in the dark.

Turn around and walk right today. Your hobbies are part of your life, but they are not your whole life. Those who hide in their garages and craft rooms or run to the gym as a form of escapism know what I'm talking about. If your hobbies become your everything, you'll stumble and fall.

The Lord has made all things, and none of them on their own are necessarily bad. I'm reminded of 1 Corinthians 10:23: "'I have the right to do anything,' you say—but not everything is beneficial. 'I have the right to do anything'—but not everything is constructive" (NIV). When your love for anything other than Him gets too big, it blocks your path. That's no good. Like a boulder in the road, your affection for other things stops you from getting through to His affection.

> For I am convinced that neither death nor life, neither angels nor demons, neither the present nor the future, nor any powers, neither height nor depth, nor anything else in all creation, will be able to separate us from the love of God that is in Christ Jesus our Lord. (Rom. 8:38–39 NIV)

God's Word is true: Nothing can separate us from His love—not even our stumbling blocks. However, our stumbling blocks can keep us from *experiencing* His love.

Have you ever been on a road trip, driving through a rugged landscape, weaving up and around mountains, bypassing boulders? Suddenly, the road bends again and you see that you're about to go straight through one of the largest mountains of all. It would be impassable except for the fact that, years ago, men with dynamite blasted through granite, shaping a tunnel clear through to the other side.

God's Word is true: Nothing can separate us from His love—not even our stumbling blocks.

Don't you know that God is dynamite—both as an adjective and a noun! He is dynamite in His awesomeness and in His ability to blow up every obstacle in our way! Those barriers, though often formed by our own two hands, can hold us back from the God who wants the fullness of our affection and attention. Our dynamite God is capable of being the dynamite that blows up each idol—each stumbling block—that separates us from Him today.

God made you for Himself. He's dynamite! Ask Him to speak clearly to your heart about any other hidden and harmful things holding you back from Him—then let Him blast through those stumbling blocks so that you might experience His loving nearness.

Dear Lord, I want to want You most of all, but I stumble over all the other things I want more. Good things, little things, big things. I am willing to cut them off and cast them down, but I need Your help. Speak to my heart today. Give me the eyes to see what idols I have made for myself, and then give me the courage to lay them at Your explosive feet. In Jesus's most powerful name I pray, Amen.

day 19

HAVE A SOBER MIND

Be alert and of sober mind. Your enemy the devil prowls around like a roaring lion looking for someone to devour.

1 Peter 5:8 NIV

OVER THE YEARS when I have asked people if they struggle with food addiction, I always receive a resounding yes. I get a similar response when I ask if they are addicted to social media or to shopping or to streaming shows and movies. When I suggest that they give up these things during our forty-day fast, I get a hallelujah chorus of Amens.

However, any time I suggest that they consider giving up alcohol, people get quiet. Real quiet. And those who don't get quiet get loud. Real loud. Defensively they exclaim, "I am not under the law, but under grace. There's nothing wrong with having a drink." They're referencing Romans 6:14: "For sin shall no longer be your master, because you are not under the law, but under grace" (NIV). But if we can't give something up for forty days, sin may still be our master.

Nobody ever tells me that this sugar fast feels legalistic, but as soon as I suggest we lay down our drinks for forty days, people accuse me of legalism.

Why? Though I agree that we are under grace to drink, why is it that we are so quick to protect our freedom to do so? What is it about alcohol that makes us protest at the thought of giving it up for forty days (or twenty-one days, if today is the day you choose to add it to the list of things you've already surrendered)?

In yesterday's reading I mentioned that the quickest way to recognize an idol in your life is to notice your response when it is taken away. If it trips you up, you've likely stumbled upon a stumbling block. **If you are convinced that you cannot forego alcohol for a few weeks, then I am convinced there's nothing you need to do more.** Matthew 19:26 makes it clear that this is impossible on your own, "but with God all things are possible." Laying down your nightly bottle of beer, glass of wine, or bourbon on the rocks may not seem possible, but with God's help it is.

This isn't about the law, friends; this continues to be a story of God's grace in our lives. This isn't a rule holding us back from fun in an attempt to be super spiritual. God gives us permission to eat and drink, but He also calls us to be on the alert and to be sober-minded. We have an enemy who loves when we are tangled up in anything that distracts us and dulls our senses. "Be alert and of sober mind," God charges us. "Your enemy the devil prowls around like a roaring lion looking for someone to devour" (1 Pet. 5:8 NIV).

It's impossible to have a sober mind when you aren't sober. Alcohol, like food and sex and getting lost online for hours, can numb our pain and dull our senses. However, more than the other addictions we've considered, alcohol dulls our senses most of all. God wants us sober because He loves us. He wants us sober as a precautionary measure, because He knows we have an enemy who is prowling around, hoping to find us distracted and, even better, a little inebriated too.

Even if we put all the spiritual stuff aside for just a moment, you probably shouldn't be drinking alcohol if you want to get the full benefit of this forty-day fast, since the sugar content is incredibly high in nearly all alcoholic beverages. Consider these facts about alcohol:

- The calories in alcohol are empty, meaning they provide no nutritional value.
- Alcohol throws off your blood sugar, interfering with your body's natural ability to regulate glucose.
- Nightly drinks disrupt other regulating hormones like insulin and glucagon.
- Even a little beer or wine can throw off the delicate balance of bacteria in your belly.[1]

There's plenty of science available to back up why it's good to fast from alcohol—whether for a season or forever—but you are still under grace to enjoy a drink if you want to. My question is, why do you want to? Or better yet, do you *want* a drink or do you *need* a drink? If you need a drink, if you need anything other than Christ to get you through each long, hard day, then I urge you to lay it down. As you abstain, you will learn that He sustains!

Nothing heightens our physical and spiritual alertness like fasting.

Nothing heightens our physical and spiritual alertness like fasting. Conversely, nothing tampers with our physical and spiritual alertness quite like alcohol. At least that is the case for me. When I fast and pray, my ears are open to hear, my eyes are open to see, and my spirit is open to discern the things of God. I'm as sober as sober can be.

God is calling you to take a sobering look at your soul's sobriety today. Are you alert? Take an honest inventory of all the ways you self-medicate and self-soothe. Don't hold anything back by clinging to your freedom in Christ as an excuse to keep doing as you please. **If the mere thought of giving up your wine causes you to whine, you might have found an idol in your life.**

Heavenly Father, You are all about freedom and flavor and fun! You're not a killjoy, standing over me with a rulebook, waiting for me to fail. I already have, time and time again. But You paid for those sins already. May my forgiven life today testify to the fact that I am truly free! And if I'm free, than I'm free to set down any and all addictions on the altar of this fast! Thank you, Jesus. In Your name, Amen.

day 20

THE WORLD'S GOODS AREN'T AS GOOD

Don't love the world's ways. Don't love the world's goods. Love of the world squeezes out love for the Father. Practically everything that goes on in the world—wanting your own way, wanting everything for yourself, wanting to appear important—has nothing to do with the Father. It just isolates you from him. The world and all its wanting, wanting, wanting is on the way out—but whoever does what God wants is set for eternity.

1 John 2:15–17 MSG

THE GOAL OF THIS FAST has been to crowd out sugar by ingesting more of God, but today we're getting honest about the things that crowd Him out. Halfway through our forty-day fast, I want you to ask yourself this question: Are the things of the world squeezing out my love for the Father? Or is my love for the Father crowding out my love for the world? You only have a limited amount of love to spend each day. How are you spending yours?

Oftentimes my husband and I look at our bank account balance with fresh eyes. After we've paid all the bills and put some money in a savings fund, we only have a certain sum left for extras. One of us suggests a new couch and the other a trip somewhere special. We consider the needs of our missionary friends who we know and love, and Christmas always seems to be right around the corner. The reality is that we have a limited amount of money, and we can't afford it all. The same is true with our affection. If we spend our energy loving things, we'll come to God spent. Flat broke and bankrupt.

These past few days we've assessed the idols in our lives—those things that we pour all our time, money, and energy into. Preeminent in our lives, they take first place in our thoughts and in our spending and in our hearts. We wake up and get out of bed in order to chase down the world's best stuff, but the world will never satisfy us because we weren't made for this world! Each day, we're seeing with new eyes that the world and the things of this world can't cut it. Not only do the world's goods not satisfy us but they also hold us back from the only One who can. That's why I'm thinking about today's verse, and how the Message translates it: "The world and all its wanting, wanting, wanting is on the way out—but whoever does what God wants is set for eternity" (1 John 2:17).

I've already talked about how the body is temporary but the soul is eternal. French Christian mystic Pierre Teilhard de Chardin put it this way: "We are not human beings having a spiritual experience. We are spiritual beings, having a human experience."[1] Don't you feel it? You are not a temporal being who can be satisfied by temporary pleasures. You are an eternal being, with a deep, insatiable hunger for eternal pleasures. Try as you might, you can't spend your life with a foot in both worlds.

The English Standard Version translates 1 John 2:15–17 this way:

> Do not love the world or the things in the world. If anyone loves the world, the love of the Father is not in him. For all that is in the world—the desires of the flesh and the desires of the

eyes and pride of life—is not from the Father but is from the world. And the world is passing away along with its desires, but whoever does the will of God abides forever.

Dear friend, don't look to debate God on this one. Of course He made this earth as a good and fertile gift, from the mango and the mandarin orange to the white cliffs of Dover and the Austrian Alps. Even children are a gift from above, coming down to us from the Father who wove them together, stitch by stitch, and placed them in our homes and our hearts. God isn't telling us to hate all the good things He made in this world. He just doesn't want us to love them more than Him, worshiping things such as food and money and clothes and fame. This world, sweet as He made it, is not our final destination. It is as brief as a breath and we're just passing through. How would our lives change if our perspective changed?

God doesn't want us to abhor the things He's made here in this world, but He doesn't want us to lust after it all, take pride in it, or allow it to steal our attention or our affection either. Our passion for the gift should never rob our passion for the Giver. Our devotion to this world shouldn't distract us from the only One worthy of our devotion. That should give us great pause!

> *Our passion for the gift should never rob our passion for the Giver.*

Throughout Scripture God likens our waywardness to adultery. That resonates with me when I pick up my phone to scroll through social media before I've taken the time to sit with Him in His Word. I know it's true when I'm tempted to buy more stuff but haven't invested my money or time in the eternal things that God values, such as orphan care and other mercy ministries. I sense it in my spirit each time I'm under stress and long for a drink instead of inviting the Holy Spirit to help me cope. I can't run in both directions at once. It's a matter of economics. If I turn to this world to get me through, I will be turning away from the One who can. It's also a matter of adultery. Adultery is the act of leaving one love for a relationship with another. This world is that other. God isn't shaming us, and I'm not trying to shame us either. But perhaps the reality of our wayward tendencies today might awake in us a *distaste* for the way we love and depend upon this world's goods just a little more than we should.

What in this world are you wanting, wanting, wanting? Are you obsessed with being thin, desired, and affirmed? Are you driven by the academic and athletic success of your children, the pride of your life? Do you spend hours on Instagram, watching home improvement shows, flipping through magazines lusting over every kitchen island and every pool overlooking Napa Valley at sunset? All those things are temporary, but you're living an eternal life now! Today is simply part of the first act in a forever musical where the eternal chorus sings, "Holy, holy, holy, is the Lord God Almighty, who was and is and is to come" (Rev. 4:8).

> *Today is simply part of the first act in a forever musical where the eternal chorus sings, "Holy, holy, holy, is the Lord God Almighty, who was and is and is to come" (Rev. 4:8).*

The Message translation speaks of our love for the world squeezing out our love for the Father. However, we're fasting now so we've turned the table. We're squeezing out the temporary pleasures of this world so that we might feast on Him forever. We're not just crowding out sugar; we're crowding out anything that has tried to crowd out our love for the Father.

Dear Lord, I want my heart to be fully devoted to You—not to this world or the things in it. Forgive me. I'm sorry it is taking me so long. Continue to show me how to love You more, because You've loved me so faithfully, and Your love never ends. Speak to me during these next twenty days. Let me hear You and see You and know You as I intentionally pull away from the things of this world and set my gaze upon eternity. In Jesus's unending name, Amen.

YOU'RE HALFWAY THROUGH

Congratulations! You've taken out sugar and perhaps some other things that have held you back from the Lord's power and presence in your life. That's the whole goal of this fast. You may have thought it was about sugar, but it's really about Jesus! More of Him, crowding out everything else. Remember, the whole point of a spiritual fast is abstaining from that which is temporary and ordinary in order to experience the One who is eternally extraordinary.

day 21

BOREDOM CAN BE
A TRIGGER TOO

Lazy people sleep soundly,
but idleness leaves them hungry.
Proverbs 19:15 NLT

WE GRAZE ON FOOD ALL DAY, misreading boredom
for hunger. And while hunger is a physical emptiness, boredom feels empty as well and we tend to get the two confused.
Perhaps, we think, *if I fill my belly, then I will feel better.* Except
overeating makes us sleepy and sleepiness makes us idle and
idleness makes us more bored and boredom makes us even
more hungry. It's a sad, lethargic cycle, and we can't break out
of it because we don't have the energy.

The New American Standard Bible translation of Proverbs
19:15 says that an idle person will "suffer hunger." *Suffering.* I
know that feeling. When I'm idle, I suffer from a false sense of
hunger—a painful urgency to fill the empty space within me,
which leads me to scour the pantry to pass the time. My favorite
translation of Proverbs 19:15 comes from the New International

Version: "Laziness brings on deep sleep, and the shiftless go hungry." *Shiftless* means lacking direction or bored and aimless. Floating here and there, without purpose, willpower, or energy—like a boat without a rudder. Can you pinpoint times in your day when you feel aimless or shiftless and mistake those feelings for hunger? Do you snack or even binge because you're bored?

The irony is that, in our boredom, too much food can end up making us sleepy. Think of Thanksgiving Day. Our family members doze on the couch after polishing off three plates of turkey, sweet potatoes, and stuffing. When we overeat, our digestive tracts get overworked. We're flooded with insulin and serotonin, which makes us drowsy. Instead of giving us energy, our digestive systems have to break down too much of the wrong food, wearing us out and lulling us to sleep. Our fatigue slows us down until we sit down, tired and bored again. As I said, it's a sad, lethargic cycle. Eventually we commit to waking up, so we turn to a hefty dose of sugar or a caffeinated beverage (or, better yet, a highly sugared *and* caffeinated drink).

Coffee and sweets combat our daily doldrums. When we ingest sugar and caffeine, our adrenal glands respond to the wake-up call like they would respond to stress—by releasing cortisol to calm us down. It's ironic. We're tired so we drink caffeine to wake us up, which triggers our bodies to release a chemical to calm us back down. We're up and down and all around, bored and stressed and eating and sleeping and drinking coffee so that we can wake up and do it all over again. Unfortunately, our adrenal glands counter each pick-me-up with another calming dose of cortisol. We're on a chemical teeter-totter and more exhausted than before!

One hand over the other, one brownie followed by more sweet tea and another cuppa joe—our adrenal glands are constantly pumping until they are so worn out they simply stop working. Depression sets in, driving us to greater exhaustion than before, and we can't cope with simple stressors without the help of cortisol. Eventually our adrenal glands aren't able to function, so we can't function. They're fatigued, so we're fatigued. They break down, so we break down. In their exhaustion they've fallen asleep, and so have we.

However, just after God tells us that the idle person will suffer hunger, He calls us to wake up once and for all. "Do not love sleep, or you will become poor; open your eyes, and you will be satisfied with food" (Prov. 20:13 NASB). Of course, this isn't merely about waking up and working hard and holding down a job so that you won't be poor. The word *poor* doesn't merely describe your financial situation; spiritual poverty is possible too—and it looks shiftless, idle, and bored. You find yourself spiritually bankrupt when you stop going to work in your faith life. That's what this wake-up call is all about. Don't fall back asleep! Wake up and go to work spiritually. Open your eyes and be satisfied with good spirit-building instead of sleep-inducing food! Friends, forget about the sugar so that you might feast on the sustaining food of Christ!

You find yourself spiritually bankrupt when you stop going to work in your faith life.

"Come to Me," God invites. "Seek Me," He implores. Stop mindlessly eating when you're bored. It is time to wake up from your slumber and actively feast on His presence. Unlike sodas and candy, He'll give you the energy you need to keep going long term—to keep running the race He has marked out for you. Hebrews 12 is the shot that rings out signifying the start of that race.

> Therefore, since we are surrounded by such a great cloud of witnesses, let us throw off everything that hinders and the sin

that so easily entangles. And let us run with perseverance the race marked out for us, fixing our eyes on Jesus, the pioneer and perfecter of faith. For the joy set before him he endured the cross, scorning its shame, and sat down at the right hand of the throne of God. Consider him who endured such opposition from sinners, so that you will not grow weary and lose heart. (Heb. 12:1–3 NIV)

Wake up! Be alert! Throw off the sin that's entangled you and run. **Open your eyes and fix them on Jesus, because He's run this race before you, and He's in your midst, running it with you now.** Don't let yourself go shiftless again. God is setting the pace. If anyone knows temptation and opposition, it's Jesus. He knows everything that causes you to grow weary and lose heart, so stay alert and stay engaged and run with Him!

Jesus, thank You for never running away from me, though I doze off from time to time. I want to wake up and run with endurance the course You've set before me. I want to be aware of the race I'm in and stay alert and strong. I know that what I'm eating isn't helping me keep up with You. Use this season of fasting to heal my body and rouse my spirit. Heal my adrenal glands and anything else that needs Your touch today. I don't want to suffer hunger another day. In the energizing name of Jesus, Amen.

day 22

SPIRITUAL AND MENTAL CLARITY

And your ears shall hear a word behind you, saying, "This is the way, walk in it," when you turn to the right or when you turn to the left.

Isaiah 30:21

I WASN'T RAISED in a fasting family or a fasting church. This idea of fasting was completely foreign to me. And yet, one day, the Lord called me to it with such clarity I couldn't resist the urge to go without food for the day.

In 1992, I was a freshman at Emerson College in Boston, Massachusetts. I was having a hard time finding other Christians at my school, so I began visiting other local colleges' campus meetings. After a while, the leaders there challenged me to start something on my own. Did I mention that I hadn't found any other Christians at my school? That's when I decided to host a Bible study for non-Christians in my dorm room. I wasn't sure who would come or what exactly I would say, but it felt like an act of obedience. The morning of the first study, I looked outside to see the Harvard rowing team gliding over the Charles River, just outside my window. Energized and alert, their eyes were set before them, their muscles tense with a synchronized purpose. I was just waking up for the day and I lacked the mental and spiritual clarity I needed for the task at hand. It was then that I decided to fast and pray, hoping that God would speak clearly to me in the hours leading up to the gathering.

The spiritual practice of fasting felt strange to me. I didn't know what exactly I was hoping to accomplish by giving up food and praying, but the direct result was clarity. It was as though God reached out, pulled off my blinders, and gave me a fresh vision for the job before me. By six o'clock that night I knew exactly how to welcome the students who showed up for the study and what I needed to share with them. It was just a simple one-day fast, but clarity came immediately.

Now here you are, twenty-two days without sugar, and I'm guessing you're likely experiencing spiritual clarity as well. How exciting! Maybe you've received revelation regarding how to serve a family in your neighborhood, a new position you're considering at work, a move across the country to be closer to loved ones, a story you've been inspired to write as a legacy to your grandchildren, a fresh way to communicate love to your spouse, or a school-district change for your children. Suddenly you have clear insight from above: "This is the way, walk in it."

While it's exciting to receive a strike of lightning-bolt clarity about something, more often the clarity that comes from fasting feels like daily insight and alertness. Slowly but surely we begin to discern what deserves a yes and what deserves a no. When we fast from sugar and feast on Scripture, we receive spiritual clarity and understanding for the path before us. Of course we do. God promises that His Word is a lamp to our feet and a light to our path—and that lamplight gives us clarity.

But there's more! I have heard my fasting friends testify that during these forty days they have not only experienced spiritual clarity but mental clarity as well.

When we fast from sugar and feast on Scripture, we receive spiritual clarity and understanding for the path before us.

Could it be that our minds work better without sugar? Could it be that we're sleeping better so our waking hours are more wakeful? Could this fast have both physiological and spiritual benefits?

Just last night, I was at a dinner party and talking with a group of friends who were all trying the latest diet craze that had them eating completely sugar-free for the first time in their lives. All three went on and on about how mentally alert they felt. "It's like I'm coming out of a fog," one said. I smiled because I knew that she was. They were all coming out from under a sugar cloud, and you are too.

Sugar and other false fillers dim our vision, but clarity is available to us when we exercise our spirits and our wills: fasting and praying, spending time in God's Word, and practicing self-control when it comes to what we eat and drink and the amount of sleep we get.

We want to hear from the Lord about which way we are to walk, and we long to clearly see His will in our daily lives. But for that to happen, we must not only ingest His Word but also consume brain food.

I've said from the start that I wouldn't be focusing on food during this fast. I know how easy it is to transfer one's obsession with unhealthy foods to an obsession with healthy alternatives. Many spiritually starving people spend their days focused solely on healthy meal planning and a workout regimen. We're not fasting from sugary food in order to fixate on healthy eating; the whole point is to fix our eyes on Jesus. He's the One who whispers instructions on where we should walk and what we should do. He's the Son who burns away the cloud cover and brings light and understanding into our days.

And so it is with caution that I encourage you to consider eating foods that are good for your brain and that help your mind work well: fish and poultry, eggs, nuts, coconuts, avocadoes, blueberries, tomatoes, broccoli, spinach, kale, and water—plenty of water. Make yourself a batch of fresh pesto or hummus to dip your veggies in this afternoon. Both are rich in Omega-3 Fatty Acids that help the brain and the body function with clarity and endurance.[1] Of course, a steady diet of God's Word is the best thing you can ingest for a clear and energizing sense of purpose each day.

We're not fasting from sugary food in order to fixate on healthy eating; the whole point is to fix our eyes on Jesus.

Again and again I remind you to feast as you fast. Let's do that now. Feast on God's Word as you pray this prayer for clarity in the days ahead.

Oh, Father in heaven, open my eyes as I open Your Word, that I may behold wonderful things from Your law. Open my ears as I open my heart to hear from You. Give me a spirit of wisdom and of revelation as I fast and pray. I humbly ask for Your clear, kind leading. In Jesus's clarifying name, Amen.

day 23

HUNGER PANGS

O God, you are my God;
  I earnestly search for you.
My soul thirsts for you;
  my whole body longs for you
in this parched and weary land
  where there is no water.

Psalm 63:1 NLT

MOST OF US aren't very good at going hungry. We're even worse at staying hungry for long periods of time. That may be why many people transition from fasting to dieting about halfway through this forty-day fast.

Here's how it happens: You're through the ugly detox stage. Physically you feel pretty good and spiritually you're closer to God than you have been in a long time, maybe ever. Wonderful! You've discovered healthier meal options and have found a rhythm to eating sugar-free. You're not so hungry anymore, not the way you were at the beginning. Your energy is up and your thinking is clear, so you've clearly gotten everything out of this fast that you're going to get. Or so you think. You're on cruise control now.

I've seen it time and again and experienced it myself. Perhaps the biggest way to slip from fasting to dieting mid-fast is learning to fill up on sugar-free foods. However, the goal in these pages and throughout these days isn't to simply detox from sugar and transfer your focus to sugar-free recipes; it's to thirst for God as though you're wasting away in a dry and parched land, to long for Him and grow in your love relationship with Him.

You are missing the point entirely if you have found a way to fast without experiencing hunger. Hunger pangs are a holy tool, reminding us that we are fasting, why we are fasting, and whom we want to be most hungry for. I love how author Bill Gaultiere said it here: "In other words, let your hunger pangs become like church bells calling you to prayer. Whenever you're hungry for food say to yourself something like, 'Jesus, you are my sweetness and sustenance. Your name is like honey on my lips. Your words are the manna that I hunger for.'"[1]

When you replace your sugary treats for sugar-free foods, you will likely lose weight and experience other health benefits. But don't you want more than that? I do! If you want a changed life, you must do more than just change your diet. Eating sugar-free may *enhance* your life, but only the Lord Himself can *transform* it. Instead, renounce sugar and replace it with a sweet and constant dependence on Christ, the Bread of Life, your sustenance. When you do that, your life will begin to change.

> *Eating sugar-free may enhance your life, but only the Lord Himself can transform it.*

It takes longer than twenty-three days to be transformed, and it requires a measure of pain—hunger pain—which is why I want you to consider how you might increase your physical hunger as a means of unleashing

your spiritual hunger. Your body is getting used to function-
ing without sugar, which is why you may be thinking you are
ready for a transition. If you want to transition, go deeper
rather than pulling back. Press into Christ rather than into
some mere diet. **Lay down your refined sugars in exchange
for His sweet refining. It's time to crank up the heat in the
crucible of this fast.**

How might you increase your physical hunger so that you
can experience greater spiritual hunger? Some people find
that eliminating other foods, such as bread and pasta, is an
easy way to crank up the intensity of this fast. Others choose
to give up breakfast completely. By waiting to eat until after
you've had a significant time with the Lord each day, you get
the intense benefits of a traditional fast each morning. Some
days that means you might have breakfast around midmorn-
ing, but other days it may not be until
noon. This practice of turning to the
Lord before turning to food will certainly turn up the heat on your fast.

Allowing yourself to go physically hungry enables your heart to grow spiritually hungry.

You'll be reminded by every empty-
belly growl that you're fasting from
sugar in order to feast on Him. Allowing
yourself to go physically hungry enables
your heart to grow spiritually hungry.
God promises that when all else fails, He
is our portion. Skip a meal or take other foods out of your diet
for the rest of this fast. See for yourself how physical hunger
ignites a deeper hunger for the One who can satisfy.

> My flesh and my heart may fail,
>   but God is the strength of my heart and my portion
>   forever. (Ps. 73:26)

I recognize how countercultural and counterintuitive it is to let yourself go hungry, but **when you push through the discomfort, you'll experience a deeper comfort than any comfort food could ever provide.** Take some time now to get quiet. Consider how much you have eaten today. Is it possible that you've simply transitioned into a sugar-free diet? Is your belly constantly full of sugar-free foods, or is it clanging like a church bell, calling you to prayer? Press into the hunger pangs as you press on through these fasting days.

In Psalm 63:8, the psalmist cries, "My soul clings to you." I have found that fasting intensifies my soul's desperation for God, causing me to cling to Him in a way I don't naturally do when I'm filled with the things of this world. What might you give up in order to intensify your soul's desperate need for God? For when you seek Him desperately, you will find Him abundantly, exceedingly, and more than you ever hoped or imagined.

Don't be afraid to get hungry; be afraid of a life that never hungers for God.

Dear Lord, I don't want to get less hungry as I fast but more hungry! Intensify my hunger for You. Use each empty-belly growl to remind me that I want You most of all. When I long for sweet refined sugars, teach me to lean into Your sweet refining. Twenty-three days into this forty-day fast, I want to want You more today than I did on day 1. Help me, Lord, to have the courage to go without, so that I might go with You! Amen.

day 24

HEALING PAST HURTS

Come to me, all you who are weary and burdened, and I will
give you rest.

Matthew 11:28 NIV

I KEEP A FILE ON MY COMPUTER that is full of the tes-
timonies people have sent me over the years as we've fasted together in community. I regularly receive messages like this one:

> During our fast, I developed a genuine self-love. As a survivor
> of childhood sexual abuse, I've struggled most of my life feel-
> ing like damaged goods. In the past, I've used food to cope and
> have made a huge mess of my health. Unfortunately, it's not
> just ruined my health, but made me miserable mentally and
> emotionally too! I am finally experiencing freedom from my
> addictions and from the negative self-talk that used to drive
> me to food. I am finally starting to experience the love of Jesus
> in my life and I am learning to completely surrender to him.

If you have been emotionally, physically, verbally, or sexually abused by a parent or a family member, a significant other
or a spouse, or anyone else in this fallen world, I am so sorry.

Truly. Even as I write these words I feel compelled to stop and pray for you. (If you haven't been abused, would you join me in praying for the men and women reading this book who have been torn apart by the sins of others?)

> *Dear Lord, before we go on with today's reading and apply Your Word to our lives, I ask that You speak truth and love to those who have been abused and are now holding this book, eager for healing. You made them and You know them. You're not finished with them yet. I humbly ask that they would open their hearts to Your healing today. Fill them up with your adoration. I pray that they grow to adore themselves because You adored them first. Gently change their thinking and their feeling and their living, so they might become healed and whole. In Jesus's redeeming name, I pray, Amen.*

Dear reader, let me give it to you straight. You are loved beyond measure and created for the explicit purpose of a safe and saving love relationship with your Creator. He made you and adores you because you are His. It is my sincere prayer that the Lord will fill you with the blessed assurance that He sees you, cares for you, and longs to redeem your hurting soul. Redeeming broken things is what He is all about. It's what He came to earth to do. He came to redeem you!

The One who knit you together in your mother's womb sent His Son to chase you down and heal you.

The One who knit you together in your mother's womb sent His Son to chase you down and heal you. Through faith you can experience Him reknitting the unraveled pieces of your life. Psalm 51:10 promises that God will make your innermost being completely new if you ask Him to. "Create in me a clean heart, O God, and renew a steadfast spirit within me" (NIV). What's more? Miracle of miracles, the reknitting doesn't happen just once. It's not a once-and-done fix. The Holy Spirit lives in you, perfecting you, healing you, and transforming you little by little as you journey toward Christlikeness and toward Christ Himself.

God didn't choose for you to be abused, but He chooses each day to redeem the abuse. He didn't want you to be hurt, but He can heal your hurt. He didn't want your mind warped by the hurtful words of others, but He can speak new words over you until you start hearing His Words rather than the words that wounded you in the past. He can and He does do all this and more when you surrender to Him as your redeemer, remaker, renewer, reknitter. All you have to do is respond to His loving invitation in Matthew 11:28, "Come to me, all you who are weary and burdened, and I will give you rest" (NIV).

He can heal any life that's been torn apart; He can fill any hole and make it whole. If you have been hurt by others and you now run to food for comfort, I know that you've found food lacking because I have too. It's not what food was made for. It's not food's job to mend you and speak truth into the lies you hear. It's God's job to comfort and fill you. He is the Great Comforter, and I'm praying that He brings you tremendous comfort and healing today and in the days ahead.

When we fast and pray, the Lord clearly and graciously shows us our soul-sadness and sin-struggles. He speaks to our hearts, tenderly and clearly, about where we've been hurt in the past and how it has caused us to behave in the present. **I've come to discover that food can be like noise, keeping us from hearing. When we set food down for a season, however, we turn the sound down and are finally able to hear the revelation of God speaking truth over our lives.**

Today I invite you to directly ask the Lord if you're running to sugar because you're running from past or present pain. It's a hard question, but one that our good God can lovingly answer. There are so many reasons why you may habitually turn to sugar. This powerful poem by Rebecca K. Reynolds lists many reasons you may run to sugar instead of the Savior.

Sugar because I'm tired—
because there's simply too much to do
and no way to do it.

Sugar because it's fast—
and I need 30 more minutes
of strength.

Sugar because I'm lonely—
because something sweet
tastes like
human touch feels.

Sugar because it's cheap—
one buck instead of five.

Sugar because I didn't plan—
didn't take time to prep
to stand against the current.

Sugar because I'm sad—
about so many things,
and for two seconds I can forget.

Sugar because I don't want to move—
and sugar sits here with me.

Sugar because I'm scared—
of what might pull me
if I were fit.

Sugar because I'm so angry—
I don't care what happens.

Sugar because I'm ashamed—
of how far I've let it go already.

Sugar because I'm addicted—
caught in a drunken cycle
of lows and highs.

Sugar because she loved by sugar—
when she wanted to give me comfort,
and I remember.

Sugar because I haven't learned to value—
what is simple and beautiful.

Sugar because I don't trust—
that manna will appear again in the morning.

Sugar because I don't believe—
I will ever adjust.

Sugar because those first three days—
are war.

Sugar because tomorrow—
tomorrow—
tomorrow I'll start.

Sugar because I never can see—
that every single today
is the first day
of the rest of a better life.[1]

Has God shown you something new during this fast? Has
He helped you understand your complicated story and some of
the age-old reasons why you turn to sugar in lieu of Him? Has
He revealed where some of your wounds came from? Perhaps

the ones that cause you to run to food as a source of comfort? If so, you now know one of your triggers. Knowledge is power. Each time you are triggered to heal the hurt with sugar, choose to respond instead by going to the One who can heal your hurt with His love. Self-medicating your pain with food keeps you from the Great Physician.

Self-medicating your pain with food keeps you from the Great Physician.

If past abuse has left you feeling unlovable, and you've learned to hide the pain behind pounds, bring those age-old hurts to the altar, and lay them there beside your sugar. Remember that giving up sugar was simply the door through which you invited the Holy Spirit deeper into your life. Now that He's up close, pressing against your hurting heart, invite Him to reknit those tattered places deep inside.

Lord Jesus, do what You are so good at doing. Knit me together again on the inside—reknit me, and renew me, and make me whole again. Fill my aching places with Your holy comfort. As I learn to rest in Your nearness, Lord, transform my thought life. Reknit my thoughts about myself. Not only does my self-loathing hurt me but it hurts You too. Teach me to love myself because You love me. Give me the eyes to see how loved I am. Fill my mind with understanding. Teach me what it means to be fearfully and wonderfully made. Though people have unmade me with their abuse, Lord, You have the authority to remake me. Mend me, Lord, and let me know the joy of being whole and wholly chosen! In Jesus's name, Amen.

day 25

GOD CARES ABOUT THE DETAILS

So we fasted and sought our God concerning this matter, and He listened to our entreaty.

Ezra 8:23 NASB

A FEW YEARS AGO I fasted from sugar as I worked on an intense writing project with a tight deadline. I'm a slow writer, so I needed clarity and focus and, perhaps, a miracle. While God answered that prayer, giving me inspiration in spades and allowing my fingers to fly over the keyboard with Scriptures and application, He was busy making improvements in my personal life as well. Though many of my hours each day were spent writing, my mind kept returning to my kids during their school days. Various needs for each one kept coming to my heart, so, as I fasted and wrote, I prayed for my children.

Oftentimes we come to a fast looking for one benefit, but the Lord decides to benefit us in other ways as well. That's what He did as I fasted. He gave me what I asked for, then addressed details that I had not invited Him into. During those days of writing and fasting, I prayed for my children and saw very specific strongholds fall away from their young lives. Grief over sin, forgiveness in broken relation-ships, breakthroughs amid learning chal-lenges . . . the details.

Oftentimes we come to a fast looking for one benefit, but the Lord decides to benefit us in other ways as well.

Similarly, we came to God twenty-five days ago with a specific prayer request, ask-ing that He do that one thing well. From that humble place, in that dependent state, we have heard from Him that sugar isn't the only thing He wants to talk to us about. In His kindness, He took us beyond what we hoped or imagined.

One by one, He has begun to reveal new details about our lives that He wants to deal with. He's getting in our personal business now, asking us to give up more things: coffee, late-night television, and online shopping too. One de-tail at a time, He's peeling back the layers of our lives like an onion. And just as peeling the layers of an onion can cause tears, so can peeling back the layers of our lives, revealing details that need God's attention. Sometimes we don't know we need Him until the other needs are peeled back revealing more. But these are good tears because they are a result of learning that God cares about all our issues—from the big and the ugly to the private and unseen.

He is sovereign over the details of our lives. Some details are overwhelming in size, such as our addictions, while others are small, such as our hidden thought lives. Marital struggles or a child's diagnosis, financial pressure and choices at work, a parent's failing health, and a possible school change for one of the kids rise to the top as God peels back layer after layer. So many details.

I'm reminded of Ezra the scribe who, after God's people were exiled to Babylon, was commissioned by King Artaxerxes to return the survivors to Jerusalem along with all the silver and gold that had been taken from the treasuries of the house of God. As Ezra prepared for the journey across the desert with the small remnant of Israelites traveling with him, he was suddenly overcome with concern for their safety.

> Then I proclaimed a fast there at the river of Ahava, that we might humble ourselves before our God to seek from Him a safe journey for us, our little ones, and all our possessions. For I was ashamed to request from the king troops and horsemen to protect us from the enemy on the way, because we had said to the king, "The hand of our God is favorably disposed to all those who seek Him, but His power and His anger are against all those who forsake Him." So we fasted and sought our God concerning this *matter*, and He listened to our entreaty. (Ezra 8:21–23 NASB, emphasis added)

Ezra brought his concern before the Lord because he knew that the details of our lives *matter* to God! What matters to us matters to Him when what matters to us is aligned with His will.

What matters to us matters to Him when what matters to us is aligned with His will.

What details concern you today? What matters deeply to you right now? Is it your work, your family, the health of a loved one, the bills that keep coming, or a specific decision that must be made this week? I have a couple of those concerns myself, but I don't want to make these decisions without God's wisdom and direction.

During the first half of this fast we focused on getting our hearts right with God, but by now God has dealt lovingly with your heart. Today you get to turn your heart and your full attention to the details that concern you. Ask the Lord to go with you and grant you wisdom and safety too. Not just for you but also for those journeying with you—your family and friends and neighbors. Take some time today to sit quietly before Him, at the foot of the throne, where He now dwells securely.

I suspect that in the past the stress caused by the details of your life caused you to run to food or some other form of consumption. But you've taken care of that now; God is God in your life. Today is the day that you take the details of your life to Him—not to sugar, not to wine, not to the gym or the scale or the mall. The only God who reigns in the heavens holds your life in the expansive palm of His hand, and He cares about all that concerns you today. **What matters to you matters to Him because you matter to Him.**

Dear Lord, You are so overwhelmingly big. I can't wrap my mind around Your vastness, Your enormous majesty, and Your complete rule over the galaxies. And yet, gentle Savior, in the person of Your divine Spirit, You also reside in the smallest space of my heart. You are in me, intimately acquainted with all that concerns me today. How kind of You to care for me as You do. Thank You, Lord. Thank You. In Jesus's name, Amen.

day 26

AS FOR ME AND
MY HOUSE...

> But if serving the LORD seems undesirable to you, then choose
> for yourselves this day whom you will serve, whether the gods
> your ancestors served beyond the Euphrates, or the gods of the
> Amorites, in whose land you are living. But as for me and my
> household, we will serve the LORD.
>
> Joshua 24:15 NIV

MANY CHRISTIANS display Joshua 24:15 on their walls and
above their mantels. Others quote it at weddings or baby dedi-
cations. Today I'd like for you to take this common Christian
saying and make it the foundation of how you live your transformed life beyond this fast.

In case you are unfamiliar with the story of Joshua, here is
a bit of background. Joshua took Moses's place as Israel ended
their forty years of wandering in the desert. Joshua was charged
with the task of leading the people of Israel into the promised land. With Joshua at the front line, the men of Israel took
the land, killed and captured the inhabitants, and settled into
their inheritance. At the end of Joshua's life, he challenged the

people to follow God and obey His commands. Joshua knew they struggled with sin and idolatry; he knew they were tempted to worship the old gods that their ancestors had worshiped, along with the gods of the people who lived in Canaan before them; but Joshua also knew that he wasn't going to live much longer, so he passionately charged them to persevere in their faith. "Throw away the gods your ancestors worshiped" he begged, "and serve the LORD" (v. 14 NIV).

When faced with a challenge that seemed overwhelming and impossible, the Israelites had a pattern of giving in to fear rather than faith. They reached for their old familiar household gods rather than the unseen, powerful, one true God. That's why Joshua delivered this charge to the next generation: "Choose for yourselves this day whom you will serve," and in the next breath, he declared, "As for me and my house, we will serve the LORD" (v. 15).

Today I want to ask you the same question. Standing on the precipice overlooking your life beyond this fast, choose for yourself—whom will you serve? The one true God or the gods who preside over present culture, who tell you to follow your appetite? Whom will you serve? And not only that but whom will your household serve? This isn't just for moms and dads and grandmas and grandpas; it's for those of you who are stepping out of your parents' home and into a home of your own for the first time. To whom will you dedicate your home and dedicate your life?

Standing on the precipice overlooking your life beyond this fast, choose for yourself—whom will you serve?

Each of us began this fast keenly aware of our sugar addiction, of our fixation on food, with the hope that it would fix us. But today we are going to turn our gaze from ourselves and our own needs to the needs of our households—to our sons and daughters, fathers and mothers, sisters and brothers, grandmas and grandpas, aunts and uncles, and to our future sons and daughters and grandchildren. Remember, we're not simply after a transformed diet but a transformed life that has the potential of transforming generations!

One of the Ten Commandments warns us that if we worship false gods, God will revisit that sin upon the next few generations (Exod. 20:5). However, if we love Him and keep His commands, He will show love to a thousand generations! Our commitment to love and obey the Lord is the most practical way that we can lead future generations to do the same! Our faith has the power to lead our future families to faith.

Our commitment to love and obey the Lord is the most practical way that we can lead future generations to do the same!

One of my favorite Bible stories that references fasting can be found in Mark 9. Here's the gist of the story: A father brought his demon-possessed son to the disciples, hoping that they would save his child from a demon's dangerous hold. After many unsuccessful attempts to call the demon out of the boy, the disciples were baffled and the father desperate. That's when Jesus walked up and asked, "What's going on?"

The father stepped up and cried:

> "Teacher, I brought my son to you, for he has a spirit that makes him mute. And whenever it seizes him, it throws him down, and he foams and grinds his teeth and becomes rigid. So I asked your disciples to cast it out, and they were not able." And he answered them, "O faithless generation, how long am I to be with you? How long am I to bear with you? Bring him to me." And they brought the boy to him. And when the spirit saw him,

immediately it convulsed the boy, and he fell on the ground and rolled about, foaming at the mouth. And Jesus asked his father, "How long has this been happening to him?" And he said, "From childhood. And it has often cast him into fire and into water, to destroy him. But if you can do anything, have compassion on us and help us." And Jesus said to him, "'If you can'! All things are possible for one who believes." Immediately the father of the child cried out and said, "I believe; help my unbelief!" And when Jesus saw that a crowd came running together, he rebuked the unclean spirit, saying to it, "You mute and deaf spirit, I command you, come out of him and never enter him again." And after crying out and convulsing him terribly, it came out, and the boy was like a corpse, so that most of them said, "He is dead." But Jesus took him by the hand and lifted him up, and he arose. And when he had entered the house, his disciples asked him privately, "Why could we not cast it out?" And he said to them, "This kind cannot be driven out by anything but prayer." (Mark 9:17–29)

The King James Version translates Jesus's response this way: "This kind can come forth by nothing, but by prayer and fasting" (v. 29). I've read many commentaries about the possible reasons most translations leave out the reference to fasting but, rather than diving into a debate about which translation is most accurate, I want to point out the role of the father's faith in this story. In verse 22, the father desperately pleaded, "If you can do anything, have compassion on us and help us." I love to consider the gentle tone of Jesus's voice as he responded, "'If you can'! All things are possible for one who believes." To which the father exclaimed, "I believe; help my unbelief!" (vv. 23–24).

Perhaps you are a parent who desperately wants to intercede for your family, but your faith feels weak. What a lesson for you to take into your home today. Do you believe? Perhaps you do, but there's still unbelief bound up in your questioning heart.

In another Gospel account of the same story, Jesus's disciple Matthew tells us that, when asked why the disciples weren't able to cast out the demon, Jesus responded, "Truly I tell you, if you have faith as small as a mustard seed, you can say to this mountain, 'Move from here to there,' and it will move. Nothing will be impossible for you" (Matt. 17:20 NIV).

Moms and dads, grandmas and grandpas, sisters and brothers, aunts and uncles, and those of you just starting to make a home on your own, choose faith. Even with faith the size of a mustard seed, you will see the Lord do tremendous things on behalf of your loved ones as you fast and pray!

Choose today whom you will serve. I know what I choose: "As for me and my house, we will serve the Lord."

Dear Lord, my household and I choose You! Over any other filler, we choose You! Before any other god, we choose You! Give me the courage to lead my family to You as I follow You by faith. I do believe; but help my unbelief! Increase my faith as I lead my family members to You. What a privilege to know You and make You known to those in my home. In Jesus's name, Amen.

day *27*

THE KIND OF FASTING GOD WANTS

This is the kind of fasting I want:
Free those who are wrongly imprisoned;
    lighten the burden of those who work
        for you.
Let the oppressed go free,
    and remove the chains that bind people.
Share your food with the hungry,
    and give shelter to the homeless.
Give clothes to those who need them,
    and do not hide from relatives who need
        your help.

Then your salvation will come like the dawn,
    and your wounds will quickly heal.
Your godliness will lead you forward,
    and the glory of the LORD will protect you
        from behind.
Then when you call, the LORD will answer.
    "Yes, I am here," he will quickly reply.

Isaiah 58:6–9 NLT

YESTERDAY WE TRANSITIONED from fasting and praying for ourselves to praying for our loved ones. Today God is calling us to look out beyond our homes, into the world.

In Isaiah 58 we read that God's people were frustrated because, despite having fasted and prayed, God seemed far away. They were eager for Him to come near to them and were frustrated that He hadn't noticed all that they were doing to seek Him. So God told them the reason they weren't finding Him was that they were going about fasting in the wrong way. "Is this the kind of fast I have chosen, only a day for people to humble themselves? Is it only for bowing one's head like a reed and for lying in sackcloth and ashes?" (v. 5 NIV). In other words, self-focused people can't garner the attention of an others-focused God!

Self-focused people can't garner the attention of an others-focused God!

Before we spend another day fasting and praying, I think we need to ask ourselves a key question: Am I fasting the right way?

The majority of people who fast do so for their own benefit. They want to hear from the Lord. They want spiritual discernment, clarity, healing, and protection. Just as the Israelites wanted to enter the promised land, we want to enter into God's promised good for our lives. Because it's hard to follow Him in such a noisy and busy world, we fast in order to pull away from the distractions. Fasting helps us hear Him clearly. That's the simple reason for fasting; it's biblical. However, as Isaiah 58 demonstrates, it's still possible to fast incorrectly.

We must be careful. Fasting isn't a magic trick. God is not a puppet whose generous strings we're pulling. **Fasting isn't a formula to get what we want but a humble invitation for God to do what He wants in our lives.** When we misuse the practice of fasting, we end up as confused as the Israelites, grumbling, "Why have we fasted? . . . Why have we humbled ourselves and you have not noticed?" (Isa. 58:3 NIV).

If you are struggling, feeling that God is not hearing you or coming to your rescue even though you've been doing this religious thing so faithfully for twenty-seven days, listen carefully. Israel asked this question:

> "Why have we fasted," they say,
>   "and you have not seen it?
> Why have we humbled ourselves,
>   and you have not noticed?"

And God answered them:

> "Yet on the day of your fasting, you do as you please
>   and exploit all your workers.
> Your fasting ends in quarreling and strife,
>   and in striking each other with wicked fists.
> You cannot fast as you do today
>   and expect your voice to be heard on high.
> Is this the kind of fast I have chosen,
>   only a day for people to humble themselves?
> Is it only for bowing one's head like a reed
>   and for lying in sackcloth and ashes?
> Is that what you call a fast,
>   a day acceptable to the LORD?" (Isa. 58:3–5 NIV)

Isaiah 58 begins with God declaring to His people loudly, like a trumpet blast, that they have been rebellious. Israel was disappointed with God, and God was disappointed with them. He basically said, "You're fasting all wrong! You think I'm happy to see you bowing and praying and focused entirely on the fasting? No! I want to see you spend your fasting days praying to me, so that you start to look like me. If that's the case, you won't be so tired and self-focused. Instead you'll be energized with a holy purpose. You're coming to me wanting something for yourself, but when you spend time with me, my top two commands will start to make sense to you: Love me with all your heart, and then love others as much as you love yourself. You're fasting all wrong because you can't get past your love of self."

Here's the lesson, friends: **We need to turn our hearts away from self-focused fasting to others-focused fasting.** Let's fast with a focus on the needs of the world. This is the heart of fasting: that we consider the heart of God.

Perhaps, as we learn to fast in this way, we will begin to see God move not only in the world but also in our own lives. Don't get me wrong. This isn't another string for us to pull on a marionette-like master. We're not changing our focus from us to others so that we can get what we've been after all along. However, when we focus on what God wants us to focus on—others—our own lives will be blessed. Take another look at Isaiah 58:6–9. It says that when we fast according to God's will, our salvation will come like the dawn, and our wounds will quickly heal. Our godliness will lead us forward, and the glory of the Lord will protect us from behind. Then when we call, the Lord will answer.

Our call is to live generously, because we are received generously.

This is not a works-based faith I'm speaking of. This generous faith-life pours out from the abundant overflow of God's kindness to us and through us! Our call is to live generously, because we are received generously. When we live and fast this way, the blessing becomes ours.

If you are missing the blessings of this life, perhaps it's because you are not doing this life properly. James 2:26 challenges that "faith without works is dead" (NASB). Stop worrying so much about what you're not eating and start feeding those in need. When you care for others as Jesus did, that's when the full joy of your salvation comes and your wounds are healed.

Oh, Lord, my God, Your love for the world amazes me. While I am coming to You with needs of my own, help me today to slow down and love those whom You love, to care for those whom You care for, to intercede for those in need around me today. Help me to catch a vision of serving others before myself, not so that my own needs are met but because You've told me to love others as I love myself. That's how I want to live during these fasting days and into all my days. Because love for others is at the center of Your heart, I want it to be at the center of mine as well. In Jesus's name, Amen.

day 28

FEED MY SHEEP

He said to him the third time, "Simon, son of John, do you love me?" Peter was grieved because he said to him the third time, "Do you love me?" and he said to him, "Lord, you know everything; you know that I love you." Jesus said to him, "Feed my sheep."

John 21:17

WRAPPING UP yesterday's lesson was hard for me. There was still so much to say. I pray, however, that yesterday's words were enough to help you transfer your fasting focus from self-seeking to others-serving.

It's not my job to tell you who to love and serve as you fast and pray, but I do want to encourage you to be still and ask God to tell you. When I have done this myself during past sugar fasts, God has led me to partner with certain ministries who are meeting the needs of oppressed people, giving them clothes and food and visiting them in their distress. What is He asking you to do? Is He calling you to take the money you are saving from that daily latte and weekly pint of ice cream and give it to a ministry caring for the homeless people in your town? Is

He calling you to support a missions organization that is digging wells for those in need of fresh water? Ask Him to show you who needs your heart and your help, your friendship and your funds.

Others will know we are Christians by our love for them. **Our strongest testimony as Christ followers in the world is how we love the world.** It is because He loved us that we love Him and because He so generously loved us that we are able to love others generously. I mentioned yesterday that our natural tendency is to love ourselves most of all, but God commands us to love Him first and foremost, others second, and ourselves last. Fasting is a time of denying ourselves so that we might grow beyond ourselves. The temptation, however, is to live self-focused lives because God focuses His love on us, but God couldn't be clearer about His desire: I love you; you love others.

Fasting is a time of denying ourselves so that we might grow beyond ourselves.

Jesus had to restate this idea to His headstrong disciple Peter three times in a row. After Jesus asked Peter, "Do you love me?" for the third time, Peter was hurt. He replied, "You know that I love you." Jesus's reply was simple. "Feed my sheep" (John 21:17).

If you love God and want to experience the miracle of a love relationship with Him in your daily life, join Him in His loving care for others. Love whom He loves, feed His sheep, and tend to His lambs and, in turn, He will feed you all that you've been hungering for and more.

> Beloved, let us love one another, for love is from God, and whoever loves has been born of God and knows God. Anyone who does not love does not know God, because God is love. In this the love of God was made manifest among us, that God sent his only Son into the world, so that we might live through him. In

this is love, not that we have loved God but that he loved us and sent his Son to be the propitiation for our sins. Beloved, if God so loved us, we also ought to love one another. (1 John 4:7–11)

When you are focused on loving the world and meeting its needs, God fills you up with His love and amazing power. Let me show you what I mean.

In January 2017, I asked those who were fasting with me to consider giving the money they were not spending on sweets to a ministry. They liked the idea and we decided to collectively support a Christian organization that was hosting an outreach program to help pregnant, impoverished women in the slums of Uganda. Together our fasting community covered the cost of an outreach to five hundred women. Our support helped to provide them with food, water, the message of the gospel, and a birthing kit, which they could take to the ministry's local birthing center to deliver their babies in a safe and sanitized environment.

Five hundred women signed up to attend the outreach event, but eight hundred pregnant women came instead. With only enough supplies for five hundred, the ministry staff started praying for God to multiply the food and medical supplies. The pastors of the local ministry began calling the names of all the women who had come, and one by one they came up to receive their kits. Amazingly, the pile did not diminish. All eight hundred women received their supplies and their meals, and many also received Christ as their Savior that day. In the end, one hundred and fifteen kits remained on the table, and an additional outreach to a new community was planned.

It was a bona fide miracle, just like the loaves and fish blessed by Jesus Himself. It was as miraculous as the widow's oil that Elisha blessed. This miracle from Jesus not only blessed hundreds of moms on the other side of the world but also our fasting community as well.

Do you want to experience the supernatural power of the God who parted the seas and set His people free from bondage in Egypt? Do you want to know the miracle-working power of a Savior who gives sight to the blind and raises the dead to life again? He is alive and well and working throughout the world. Join Him by feeding His sheep! Each time you're tempted to overfeed yourself, stop and pray, *God, whom would You have me feed today? I don't need more.*

He is alive and well and working throughout the world. Join Him by feeding His sheep!

Many of us overeat because we're bored with our self-focused lives. Let's choose instead to turn our attention to those who are physically hungry, and let that grow in us a spiritual hunger like nothing we've ever known before!

Dear wonder-working Savior, I do love You. Help me to take my eyes off myself and put them on those who are hungry and in need throughout the world, throughout my city, and even in my close circle of friends and family. Holy Spirit, inspire me and show me whom I am to love today. Show me how to love as I fast and pray for the benefit of others. In Jesus's loving name, Amen.

SHARE GOD'S LOVE WITH OTHERS

During this time of fasting, let me encourage you to choose a practical way that you might generously share the love of God with those in need. This fast isn't about you, it's about Christ in you—and ultimately He wants to love others through you. Don't worry about your own needs right now. **Trust God to take care of you as you make yourself available to care for others.**

Tally up the money you're saving from cutting out sugar and send it to a ministry that's sharing the Good News throughout the world. Sponsor a child through an organization like Compassion International.[1] Spend some of your fasting days serving with a local ministry. Or, if you would like to join me in giving to The Lulu Tree,[2] you can find out more at 40daysugarfast.com.

Fasting is a common religious practice, but remember that "religion that God our Father accepts as pure and faultless is this: to look after orphans and widows in their distress" (James 1:27 NIV). **You can share the Good News with others by sharing your love and resources.** Make giving an important part of your fasting these next eleven days.

day 29

DITTO

In the same way, the Spirit helps us in our weakness. We do not know what we ought to pray for, but the Spirit himself intercedes for us through wordless groans. And he who searches our hearts knows the mind of the Spirit, because the Spirit intercedes for God's people in accordance with the will of God.

Romans 8:26–27 NIV

DURING THE PAST FEW DAYS I have been talking about how God wants to use you to help meet the needs of others, but today it's my joy to remind you that your needs aren't going unrecognized by the Father. Romans 8:26–27 promises that the Spirit is interceding for us, and then just a few verses later, we're told, "Christ Jesus is He who died, yes, rather who was raised, who is at the right hand of God, who also intercedes for us" (v. 34 NASB). Both God's Son and His Spirit are speaking directly to the Father on our behalf today. Amazing! What's more? Their prayers for us are in complete harmony with God's perfect will for our lives.

Recently I have taken to praying a simple faith-filled prayer: *Ditto.* In other words, I bow my head and agree with whatever it is that Jesus and the Spirit of God are praying on my behalf. I throw out a hearty, "What He said," followed by an "Amen."

Marriage is hard, parenting is hard, life in this fallen world is just plain hard and, at times, I simply don't know how to pray—for myself or others. That's when I remember that "the Spirit himself intercedes for us through wordless groans" (Rom. 8:26 NIV). I imagine the Son leaning over the armrest of His father's throne, talking quietly to Him about what concerns me and my loved ones today.

Psalm 138:8 says, "The LORD will accomplish what concerns me" (NASB). Though I can't get my mind around all that is on my heart today, Jesus knows, He cares, and He is working it out. Though I don't know how to pray or what to pray, He does—in perfect alignment with the Father's sovereign and loving will for my life. Oh, what peace that affords me when the winds blow hard and the waves crash over me! The Son, who calmed the seas with a word, is speaking a word on my behalf into the Father's ear.

> *The Son, who calmed the seas with a word, is speaking a word on my behalf into the Father's ear.*

While you came to this fast wanting to get a handle on sugar and to break its hold on you, I imagine you have other deep concerns on your mind today—needs that you might not even be able to articulate right now.

Perhaps you're in desperate need of saving in a relationship, one that has put you in physical or emotional pain. Maybe you've wandered so far from God in an area of your life, you can't imagine breaking away from where you are and coming back to Him. How do you wrap a prayer around such heartache? Maybe it's your child or your spouse who has wandered away from both God and your family, and the heart pain is so immense that it's left you groaning or even mute. Let me remind you that the God who is able to save you, can save you completely.

> Therefore he is able to save completely those who come to God through him, because he always lives to intercede for them. (Heb. 7:25 NIV)

Jesus died so that you could live with the Father eternally. Now Jesus lives to bring you to the Father prayerfully. Praise Him for His continued care and add your Amen to His continued prayers on your behalf. Agree with His good will for your life, and rest, for nothing is too difficult for Him. Nothing that concerns you today is too big for God. If you are tempted to disagree, remember Genesis 18:14, where the Lord asked Abraham this rhetorical question: "Is anything too difficult for the LORD? At the appointed time I will return to you, at this time next year, and Sarah will have a son" (NASB).

Jesus died so that you could live with the Father eternally. Now Jesus lives to bring you to the Father prayerfully.

Though odds and age were stacked against Abraham and his wife, God miraculously enabled them to conceive. Centuries later, Jesus looked into the eyes of His disciples and said, "With man this is impossible, but with God all things are possible" (Matt. 19:26).

Even back before God revealed Himself to Abraham, Job confessed, "I know that You can do all things, and that no purpose of Yours can be thwarted" (42:2 NASB). Isn't that why we humble ourselves to pray this simple prayer? *Ditto.* Because we desire God's purpose above and beyond our own. Jesus and the Holy Spirit are interceding for us. What a relief!

Dear Father, You are on the throne and over all, and Your Spirit and Your Son are with You, interceding for me today. I humbly bow my head and lift my grateful Amen. Thank You for being so intimately acquainted with all that concerns my heart today. By the power of the Holy Spirit and in the name of Jesus, Amen.

day 30

AT THE TABLE WITH JESUS

He brought me to the banqueting house, and his banner over
me was love.

Song of Solomon 2:4

WHEN I WAS A CHILD, I sang a simple chorus in Sunday
school that was based on the verse above. The song filled my
imagination with thoughts of family, belonging, and good food
too. I imagined that every meal in heaven would be like Thanksgiving, with God at the head of the table. I liked to think about
what heavenly desserts would be like, and I wondered how
many people could fit at the table with us.

Those of you who also love good food and fellowship will
understand my affection for Song of Solomon 2:4. Though
other Scriptures have added to my growing understanding
of heaven, I continue to love the thought of God intimately
preparing a place for me, one that includes a banquet hall, a
table, and good food. Above that long, inclusive table hangs
one large, sweeping sign proclaiming God's love. For me, however, simply having a seat at that table is sign enough that I
am loved.

The first chapter of Song of Solomon gives us another picture of God's intimate love for us. We're told: "The king has brought me into his chambers" (1:4). A castle's chambers are the innermost rooms where the family dwells, and I like to think that God invites us into the most intimate parts of *His* house. That's where we belong. That's the home that He's prepared for us, not a brand-new mansion just down the street for each new convert, as I always imagined, but a room in God's own family home.

During the writing of this book, my husband and I took our first trip to Israel. On the banks of the Sea of Galilee, in the village of Capernaum, we stood beside the ruins of an ancient Jewish home. Its outer walls were long and made of stones, forming one massive square. Inside the home were smaller rooms. Looking carefully, we could clearly see how the home had originally been divided into four large living spaces, and then subdivided each time a child or a grandchild took a wife and started a family of their own. They didn't build a new house when new additions to the family arrived; they prepared a new place within the family house. In the same way, we've all been invited into God's household through faith. And Christ, the firstborn of many brothers and sisters, went into His Father's house ahead of us to prepare places for us to dwell with Him. Dividing His inheritance, Christ made a place for each one of us in those innermost chambers, and He set a seat at His table too.

This idea of living with God in His home changes everything for me as I consider the family table He invites us to. In a family there's always someone in the kitchen. If there's bread to be made, might Christ and I be making it together then breaking it together? And if we're preparing a family meal together, won't we talk intimately as family members do? Why else is

He so passionate about sharing his innermost chambers with me? Suddenly the banqueting table represents so much more. My imagination is more alive than ever; I hear the sound of laughter and storytelling rising in our forever-home with its many, many, many rooms.

If Christ died to save me for an eternity with Him, I imagine He wants to spend it intimately with me. Why wouldn't He want me to enjoy that sweet intimacy now as well? If I am going to enjoy face-to-face conversations with my Savior each day in eternity, what should my prayer life look like today? It's a good question to ask when we're fasting and praying. Fasting makes me quiet and gives me ears to hear. It intensifies my desire to talk with the One I'll be dining with one day.

If Christ died to save me for an eternity with Him, I imagine He wants to spend it intimately with me.

Will there be a large banquet table in heaven? I imagine so! Will there by an immense house with many rooms? I hope so! What will it be like to sit around the table with the Father and the Holy Spirit and the Son? I can only imagine. But I'll tell you this: I'm not going to wait to start enjoying it. I'm committed to enjoying His fellowship right now!

Use these fasting days to talk intimately with the One who intimately invites you into His family and into His home. Pray your way through these fasting days. **What's fasting without prayer? Why, I think it's merely going hungry.** Here's my question to you: Have you been enjoying His nearness during this fast? This isn't merely a physical detox; it's an opportunity to draw nearer to One with whom you will spend eternity. Don't wait for heaven to talk intimately with the Father and the Son. You're family now.

Dear Jesus, thank You for coming to earth and calling me to faith and making a way for me to come back to the Father. You generously gave Your life on earth, rose again, then went on ahead to prepare Your heavenly home for me to join You there. I'm so excited to be with You one day—to talk with You and laugh with You and share meals with You around that banquet table. Yes, that thought alone testifies to the fact that I am loved! I love You too and am so thankful that I can prayerfully talk with You right now! Amen.

day 31

PRAYING FOR HEALING

If my people who are called by my name humble themselves,
and pray and seek my face and turn from their wicked ways,
then I will hear from heaven and will forgive their sin and heal
their land.

2 Chronicles 7:14

A FEW YEARS AGO, I received a letter from a woman
letting me know that during our sugar fast she received her
hearing back. Though she had been deaf for a decade, she was
now suddenly and miraculously able to hear again. Scriptures
and Bible stories flooded my mind: Stories where the blind were
given sight and the paralyzed were invited to stand. Stories of
women and men, young and old, who were raised from sickness and death and given a new lease on life. I remembered the
story of the ten lepers whom Jesus healed and how only one of
them ran back to thank Him. With that thought swirling in my
head, I kneeled down and praised God for healing this woman
so miraculously.

Despite having been privy to this bona fide miracle, when
the next online sugar fast rolled around the following year,

I was nervous about encouraging people to ask the Lord for healing. I had lost my boldness. *What if God doesn't show up in miraculous ways?* I wondered. *What then?* While I believed that He was still able to heal any and every disease or disorder, I also knew that He doesn't always choose to do it in our way, in our time, or sometimes at all.

Around that time, I ran into the missions pastor at my church. I hadn't seen him for half a year since he'd been moving back and forth between home and the hospital, battling cancer for six strenuous months. I thought of him regularly, and each time he came to mind, I asked God to heal him. When I spotted him in the church lobby that Sunday morning, I practically ran to him. I was eager to hear how he was doing and how the Lord was answering my prayers. "I've been praying for you," I said.

Pastor Dave smiled. He was thinner than he had been the last time I saw him; his lips were dry, and his eyes wet. "I'll tell you how I have learned to pray recently," he offered instead of a prognosis. Then he leaned down, as though sharing a secret with a child. I knew in that moment that I was the student and he was the teacher, so I listened hard. My pastor went on, "I've learned to ask the Lord for whatever sort of healing He wants for me. I simply pray, *Lord, You know I have cancer and that I would like for You to heal me, but I want You to know that I'll take whatever healing You want for me. I'm hoping for my body but perhaps You want to heal my thinking or my speaking or my relationships. Heal whatever You want to heal in me today.*" With that, Pastor Dave smiled, turned, and walked slowly into the sanctuary.

His prayer made sense to me and lifted the weighty expectation that God's healing needs to be in accordance with our will. I went home and invited my fasting community to ask God to heal them during our forty days of fasting. *Lord,* we prayed individually, *You know I have this particular illness and You know all about that relationship that needs healing too. But I want You to heal me however You want to heal me. Heal my cells and heal my thinking and heal my spending and heal my family relationships too. Bring them all into submission with Your will for my life these forty days! In Jesus's name, Amen.*

After that year's fast was over, I received half a dozen letters about marriages that had been miraculously restored and children who had been miraculously healed of illnesses. I don't know if these healings were in response to specific prayers, or simply the result of a loving and sovereign God responding to the cries of those who, by faith, asked Him for whatever healing He wanted for them. When you believe in the goodness of a sovereign God—and the sovereignty of a good God—your faith in Him transcends the specifics of your prayer requests. Your desire for the Healer precedes all desire for the healing. I'm often reminded, when I am praying for specific issues, that the woman whose hearing was restored had likely not been fasting and praying for her hearing to be restored. That was her prayer long ago. She was simply fasting from sugar so that she might feast on the Healer, and His good plan for her was to open her ears.

When you believe in the goodness of a sovereign God— and the sovereignty of a good God— your faith in Him transcends the specifics of your prayer requests.

Should we pray specifically? Yes. Absolutely. Jesus said that we don't have because we don't ask. He told us that we can, by faith, point to a mountain and tell it to move and it will move! Sickness is a mountain, an unfaithful and unrepentant spouse is a mountain, a child who has gone astray is a mountain, an ailing parent's dementia is a mountain, scoliosis is a mountain, cancer is a mountain. We have been given the authority of the One who made the mountains to command them to move, but we also know that our prayers won't thwart the good purposes of a good God!

Today I invite you to pray specifically, boldly believing God will answer according to His good and overarching will.

While our focus these forty days is on the supernatural work that happens in our spiritual lives as we fast, I have come to see that physical healing often takes place when people cut out refined sugars. Inflammation in joints and muscles and common aches and pains often miraculously disappear when we fast from sugar. Headaches, acne, insomnia, restless legs syndrome, and diabetes do too. I often receive testimonials of emotional and psychological healing as well. Anxiety, depression, and debilitating fear diminish when sodas, candy, and highly sugared treats are laid at the feet of the Great Physician.

> *Fasting is going without that which you thought you needed in order to experience the power and presence of the One you need most of all.*

If ever there is a time to pray for healing, I believe it is while one is fasting. Your body is primed and ready for a healing touch. Fasting is going without that which you thought you needed in order to experience the power and presence of the One you need most of all. Let Him heal you. With a hungry heart and a growling belly, boldly approach the throne of grace, trusting in the resurrecting power of the Great Physician and His ability to miraculously heal what most needs healing today.

Thank You, God, for knowing me. You are well aware of all that concerns me medically and relationally today. I invite You, Lord, to heal me—whatever that means to You. You know just what I need and I trust You. For my good and for Your glory I ask all of this in the name of Jesus Christ, Amen.

day 32

WAKE UP!

Rise up, you women who are at ease, hear my voice;
    you complacent daughters, give ear to my speech.
In little more than a year
    you will shudder, you complacent women;
for the grape harvest fails,
    the fruit harvest will not come.
Tremble, you women who are at ease,
    shudder, you complacent ones;
strip, and make yourselves bare,
    and tie sackcloth around your waist

Isaiah 32:9–11

WITH A LITTLE OVER A WEEK LEFT to fast and pray, you must not rest on the laurels of what God has already done. The walls that He brought down in the early days of this fast were but outer walls. All that He's said and done was just the groundwork for that which He's about to do in you. He is inside the gates now, closer than ever, but parts of you are still walled off, hidden in an inner room somewhere. The days that remain are crucial because it is often in the final days of a fast that

God tears down your most intimate defenses. The early days of your fast focused on the outer walls of your physical detox, but these last days secure your spiritual transformation. If you grow complacent now, the private and mostly unseen walls will remain standing and secure, and they will continue to separate you from the faith and freedom you most desire.

Don't let complacency hold you back from taking the final blows that can bring down the most stubborn walls. Don't lose the red-hot fire that set you on course thirty-two days ago. Stay the course. If you find that you're fasting out of habit today, don't give in these last few days. Recommit. Don't be lazy; be vigilant! Don't fast out of habit, as though fasting is merely a physical exercise of your will. Remember what God has already done and get hungry to see Him do more!

> *Remember what God has already done and get hungry to see Him do more!*

The fire that you felt at the start of this fast must not cool or you'll enter your post-fast life lukewarm. While you may think that lukewarm is better than how you were before this journey began, don't be fooled. Scripture tells us that lukewarm is never okay.

I love the letters God inspired the apostle John to write to the early Christian churches, recorded for us in the book of Revelation. If we are humble enough, we can admit the same tendencies toward complacency in our lives today. To the church in Laodicea, God said: "I know your deeds, that you are neither cold nor hot; I wish that you were cold or hot. So because you are lukewarm, and neither hot nor cold, I will spit you out of My mouth" (Rev. 3:15–16 NASB).

Even if we have put our faith in Christ and are part of His church, we can still fall asleep in our faith. Even if we sit our bodies down in a pew on Sundays, our hearts can still be complacent most hours of every day. Fasting friends, don't fall asleep during the final days of this fast. Wake up! Let's swing open wide the innermost doors of our hearts and pray, *Jesus, I want more! I want to hear You! I want to get lit up and red hot and fired up. I've grown satisfied with being unsatisfied, and I don't want to live that way any longer.*

Revelation isn't the only place in Scripture where God expresses displeasure about spiritual complacency. He also spoke words of warning through the prophet Zephaniah: "At that time I will search Jerusalem with lamps, and I will punish the men who are complacent . . ." (1:12). Let me ask you, are you still hiding parts of your life in the dark? Because a time is coming not only in Jerusalem but throughout the whole earth, when the Son of God will shine His light into the dark recesses of every heart and in every home the world over! I cannot say what that punishment will be, in light of God's grace to those who have believed, but I have no doubt that Jesus wants more for us than a sleepy faith that rests on the laurels of "I believe."

If we believe Jesus is the Son of God who came to set us free from sin and shame and an eternity separated from the Father, then our faith lives should be red hot! We have been redeemed at a cost so high only the blood of our Savior could cover it all. English evangelist Leonard Ravenhill asked this pointed question: "Are the things you are living for worth Christ dying for?"[1] That's the wake-up question. If we truly believe we have been bought with the precious blood of God's own Son, how can we remain lukewarm? The Father will spit from his mouth a faith that is tepid.

Oh friends, there is only one week of fasting left, and I don't want you to miss out! If this fast was only about muscling the willpower to forego sugar, nothing's going to change in your

life come day 41. However, if your faith gets hot—really hot—
then the impurities in your life are going to rise to the surface.
Sugar addiction and every other sin tendency will come to the
top and the Lord will sweep it off, like a refiner removing the
dross from precious metal. You are precious to the Lord! So
precious that He gave His Son so that you might live! What
are you living for? How are you living? Are you shining for the
Lord, or are parts of you still in the dark, walled off behind an
inner door somewhere?

At the end of God's letter to the church of Laodicea, He
said:

> Behold, I stand at the door and knock; if anyone hears My voice
> and opens the door, I will come in to him and will dine with
> him, and he with Me. He who overcomes, I will grant to him
> to sit down with Me on My throne, as I also overcame and sat
> down with My Father on His throne. He who has an ear, let him
> hear what the Spirit says to the churches. (Rev. 3:20–22 NASB)

We often take this passage out of context for non-Christians,
but these words are an invitation, a knocking on the door of
the church, a letter to believers. **Don't become complacent;
open the innermost door of your heart and let Jesus have
full access to your life!**

*Dear Lord, I don't want to fool myself and believe that I have
gotten everything out of this fast. If I'm still fasting, then I'm
still praying, and if I'm still praying, then You're still listening. I want to listen too. Speak to me, Lord. Speak to me about
anything and everything that remains between us. I want those
final walls demolished, so that You might go deeper in me than
ever before. In Jesus's refining name, Amen.*

day 33

BRICK BY BRICK

The wise woman builds her house,
But the foolish tears it down with her own hands.

Proverbs 14:1 NASB

ON THE THIRD DAY OF OUR FAST, I told you to expect
the Lord to bring down some nasty strongholds in your life—
with sugar chief among them. Since then, the beloved Sunday
school hymn about Joshua and Jericho and walls tumbling down
has been playing on loop in my mind. This morning, as I opened
up the Bible to the book of Proverbs, my eyes fell upon a warning: "Like a city whose walls are broken through is a person who
lacks self-control" (Prov. 25:28 NIV). *Oh my!* I thought, *I want
some walls to fall, but not as a result of my own foolish, undisciplined
life.* In that moment I realized a simple fact: Walls are going to
fall either way, but which walls and by whose hands they come
down is entirely up to me.

There are bad walls—we've called them strongholds—but
there are good walls too. Our job is to yield to the good structures that the Lord has protectively placed around us, as we
continually invite Him to bring down the strongholds that have

held us back from His promises and from His promised land. So often, we tear down the wrong walls, the walls that God lovingly erected to safeguard us within.

Looking back over my life, I see the walls He hemmed me in with: commands and instructions about everything from sexual purity and honoring my parents to not gossiping. Even today I see Him attempting to build a safeguard around me, telling me through His Word to not give in to envy. When

Our job is to yield to the good structures that the Lord has protectively placed around us.

I remain within these good walls, my life is good. But it takes ongoing submission to God's will over my will each day for me to stay planted in Him.

All throughout the Scriptures God instructs us about how to pray and how to rest and how to serve and how to eat and how to live. Our natural tendency, of course, is to choose which of His instructions we will submit to, which of His walls we will allow to remain. For the most part, we do what we want and follow our own passions. Brick by brick, we choose which walls stay up and which come down. We choose who we will date, what we will look at online, if we will be generous with our time and resources, which thoughts we will take captive and which ones will hold us captive, how much we will drink, if we will read our Bible, and if we will spend more money than we make. With one hand over the other, we tear down the protective structures God has placed around us and eventually the walls come tumbling down.

What does this have to do with our forty-day sugar fast? We're denying ourselves what we hunger for as a means to submit our appetites to God. In the same way, we must deny our impulses to build the life that we want over the life that Christ died to give us. The bending of our wills concerning what we eat is an exercise in submission as much as it is in self-control. More so, in fact, for submission is ultimately about God-control. God controlling our lives, God controlling our compulsions, God controlling our tongues, God controlling the placement of each wall that holds us in or holds us back.

The more I think about the various walls that need to come down in my life, the more I sense God calling me to consider the good walls I've torn down and the ones I've constructed in their stead. Some of the strongest, saddest walls that have held me back from God's plans for my life weren't erected by a figurative Jericho but by my own two hands. **Choices I made over time turned into habits that turned into strongholds.** Even what we eat, over time, can become a wall if we're not careful. Our choices become barriers that hold us back from health, wholeness, and freedom.

Whether we understand His boundaries or not, agree with them or not, or want them or not, they are for our protection. Psalm 16 sings this truth over us: "LORD, you alone are my portion and my cup; you make my lot secure. The boundary lines have fallen for me in pleasant places; surely I have a delightful inheritance" (vv. 5–6 NIV).

God doesn't simply rebuild broken walls; He resurrects broken lives.

Today consider which walls you've foolishly torn down. Which of God's instructions that work like a protective structure have you demolished? Repent of the life you've built outside of those boundaries. God is faithful to restore what you've torn down. God doesn't simply rebuild broken walls; He resurrects broken lives. "I will build you up again, and you, Virgin Israel, will be rebuilt. Again you will take up your timbrels and go out to dance with the joyful" (Jer. 31:4 NIV).

Submit to His rebuilding!

God Almighty, Your Word is the structure I want to abide within. I am sorry I've lived undisciplined, tearing down what You've created in lieu of what I want. Today I choose to want what You want for me. Rebuild my life upon the firm rock of my salvation, Jesus Christ. Hide me within Your protective walls so that I might shout from its ramparts just how pleasant it is to dwell in the land You've given me. Thank You for Your ongoing, rebuilding grace. Because of Jesus, Amen.

ONE WEEK TO GO!

With one week of fasting left, it's time to start considering if a sugar-free lifestyle beyond these forty days would be good for you. Do you feel physically healthier, mentally clearer, emotionally more stable, and spiritually stronger? Are you less irritated with your loved ones and hungrier for the Word? **Once the stronghold of sugar comes tumblin' down, a sugar-free structure may help to keep you safe and free.**

Recently my pastor was talking about the structures God puts in our lives to keep us safe. He likened God's laws to the bars that hold you in on a roller coaster ride. That protective structure isn't intended to get in the way of having fun but, instead, to make it possible to have fun! Likewise, structuring the way you eat doesn't have to stop you from enjoying food. A protective safety structure might actually hold you in securely and free you up to enjoy all aspects of your life more fully!

You don't need to make the decision today, but give it some thought as you fast and pray.

day 34

REMEMBER!

When the disciples reached the other side, they had forgotten to bring any bread. Jesus said to them, "Watch and beware of the leaven of the Pharisees and Sadducees." And they began discussing it among themselves, saying, "We brought no bread." But Jesus, aware of this, said, "O you of little faith, why are you discussing among yourselves the fact that you have no bread? Do you not yet perceive? Do you not remember the five loaves for the five thousand, and how many baskets you gathered? Or the seven loaves for the four thousand, and how many baskets you gathered?"

Matthew 16:5–10

YOU STILL HAVE ONE WEEK LEFT to fast and pray, but today's Scripture is making me think of day 41. **When this fast is over, will you remember how God filled you to overflowing as you spent time with Him? Or will He need to keep working miracles on your behalf to keep your attention?**

At the beginning of Matthew 16, Jesus had just arrived on the other side of the Sea of Galilee after feeding four thousand men. As soon as He stepped off the boat, He was approached by a group of Pharisees and Sadducees bent on testing Him. They asked Him to show them a sign to prove that He was the Son of God, the Messiah. Of course, Jesus wasn't after followers who needed proof of His deity; He wanted (and still wants) faithful followers who believe through faith and not visual evidence. Jesus responded to their request with this: "An evil and adulterous generation seeks after a sign; and a sign will not be given it, except the sign of Jonah" (Matt. 16:4 NASB). Only after His death and resurrection would it become clear that Jesus was referring here to His own resurrection. Jonah was swallowed up in a watery grave for three days and then spit out on the shore. Jesus was in the grave for three days before God resurrected Him. Jesus knew that even after He gave the ultimate sign of His deity, His resurrection, the religious leaders would still not believe, so He walked away from them and got back into the boat with His disciples.

Can you imagine Jesus in that moment? He left the Pharisees and Sadducees and their faithless request for miracles, and was sitting with his followers who had just watched Him feed thousands of people with a few fish and a couple loaves of bread. Unfortunately, His disciples had already forgotten that miracle and were grumbling that they had forgotten to bring bread with them. That's when Jesus said, "O you of little faith, why are you discussing among yourselves the fact that you have no bread? Do you not yet perceive? Do you not remember the five loaves for the five thousand, and how many baskets you gathered? Or the seven loaves for the four thousand, and how many baskets you gathered?" (Matt. 16:8–10). Even Jesus's closest companions required sign after sign for their faith to remain engaged.

As we draw near the end of this fast, purpose in your heart to remember the faithful way God has provided for you. When you remember God's past faithfulness, you are more prone to stay faithful to Him. If He's revealed His faithful love to you these forty days, revel in it! Don't simply move on with the hope of living different. Continue living each day with Him and you will live differently. Keep on going.

When you remember God's past faithfulness, you are more prone to stay faithful to Him.

In the passage that began today's reading, the disciples exclaimed that they had forgotten to pack bread for their journey. It makes me laugh. Jesus wanted to take His friends deeper, teaching them more about Himself and the Father's love, but they were stuck on yesterday's lesson. They didn't remember what God had done to sustain them in the past.

Likewise, at the end of their forty years of wandering in the desert, Moses cautioned the children of Israel to remember the Lord's provision to them during their time in the desert. God provided food in the form of manna so that they did not go physically hungry. Moses's warning to the Israelites concluded with this reminder: "Man does not live by bread alone, but man lives by every word that comes from the mouth of the LORD" (Deut. 8:3).

Isn't that what you've been learning too—that it isn't food that ultimately sustains you but God and His Word? Your body may be learning that it feels healthier physically when you're not eating sugar, but your spirit is learning to feast on God and on every word that comes from His mouth. He's faithfully filled you with His Spirit and provided you with everything you need during this fast and beyond. **He has proven Himself faithful; now you must remain faithful.**

Don't forget the way God miraculously fed you from His own table as you fasted from the sweetest treats this world has to offer.

Let's purpose in our hearts to remember the lessons He has already taught us these past few weeks so that He might teach us new and wonderful things about Himself. Psalm 119:18 invites us to pray, "Open my eyes that I may see wonderful things in your law" (NIV). God is eager to open our spiritual eyes to new, mind-blowing realizations about life with our Savior. He bids us, "Call to me and I will answer you and tell you great and unsearchable things you do not know" (Jer. 33:3 NIV).

He has proven Himself faithful; now you must remain faithful.

There is so much more life to be had when you walk with Christ each day. Make it your goal to remember what He's already revealed so that you might be ready for more.

Holy Spirit, help me to remember what I've learned so that I don't have to go back and relearn these same lessons again and again. I'm eager to learn more from You now. Open my eyes and allow me to see wonderful new things in Your law, and open my ears so that You can tell me all the unsearchable things that I do not yet know. And when I forget, for I will forget sometimes, gently remind me again. In Jesus's patient name, Amen.

day 35

ONCE YOU'RE FREE,
YOU'RE FREE TO SHARE

While they were worshiping the Lord and fasting, the Holy Spirit said, "Set apart for me Barnabas and Saul for the work to which I have called them."

Acts 13:2

GOD OPENS YOUR SPIRITUAL EARS when you fast. That is why, as I wrote this guide to accompany your fast, I asked Him to speak clearly to you. The Bible is filled with stories of people receiving a clear word from the Holy Spirit as they fasted and prayed.

Perhaps as you have been worshiping the Lord these past few weeks, the Spirit of God has spoken directly to you. Maybe you've heard Him speak about something in your life that needs to be *set aside* for a specific work that God has called you to do. Maybe He's calling you to fill a volunteer position in the church or maybe He's calling you to step down from a commitment you've made. Or it could be that He's whispered "stay" as you've fasted and prayed with open hands and a broken marriage. Sometimes He calls you to say yes and other times He calls you to say no, which is why you need to carefully listen for His still small voice.

Whether He's calling you to host an outreach event in your neighborhood (perhaps an Easter egg hunt or a Sunday brunch) or to be more present and available to your children and spouse (putting down your phone at the table and opening the Word together), God is passion- *God speaks to* ate about the redemptive work in the lives of His people. I don't know the particulars of *us intimately* what God's Holy Spirit is saying to you, but I *because we are* have to believe He is speaking, because that's *intimately His.* what He does. I said it early on, but I'll say it again: The same God who saves also speaks. God speaks to us intimately because we are intimately His.

He has good plans for our lives and good works for us to do. Ephesians 2:10 tells us, "For we are his workmanship, created in Christ Jesus for good works, which God prepared beforehand, that we should walk in them." If God lovingly fashioned us for good works, preparing us for them and them for us, then He is kind enough to help us find those specific good works. He is not an elusive God, nor a far-off God, but a clear-speaking and present God who gives us the guidance of His Spirit and the illuminating light of His Word.

Still, sometimes I feel completely in the dark about what God would like me to do. One prayer I pray regularly, especially as I fast and ask the Lord for clarity, is this: *God, I'm not very smart, but I have a "here I am, send me" heart. So You've got to make it clear, Lord. You've just got to! Tell me what You want me to do and I'll do it. But please, please don't make it hard for me to understand because my heart's desire is to do Your will. In Jesus's clarifying name, Amen.*

Today, as you worship the Lord with fasting and prayer, invite Him to speak with you clearly, as with a friend. Ask Him what He is calling you to do. Now that your fast is drawing to a close, you're being freshly commissioned to do His work. After all, He didn't send just Saul and Barnabas out to do the work of the gospel; He has sent us all out. Before Christ ascended into heaven, He commissioned all believers to go and tell the world about Him: "Go therefore and make disciples of all nations, baptizing them in the name of the Father and of the Son and of the Holy Spirit" (Matt. 28:19). **Those who have experienced the bondage-breaking power of God are called to share the source of such power with those still held captive.** Every person who believes in Jesus has been charged with the clear command to go and preach the good news of salvation and freedom through Christ.

Sugar has lost its seat on the throne of your life, and Christ is securely seated there now. It's time to get going. **Your Savior King has good works for you to do and good news for you to proclaim. That is your mission and your commission.** God has an assignment for you to do. Your job now is to pray about the details of that assignment.

Once you have been called to faith, you're called to share your faith, which often looks like simply sharing your life. Early on, the disciples had to leave their homes *Christ has set* and go to the far reaches of the world. There *you free, which* are still missionaries going to the unreached corners of the globe today, but you can also *sets you free to* be called to reach those right where you are. *share Him!* When you share the details of your saved and redeemed life with those in your midst, you're sharing a beautiful picture of redemption.

The Lord has delivered you from sugar shackles, and you're no longer running to false fillers in your life. You are a transformed, living, breathing testimony of what God can do. **Christ has set you free, which sets you free to share Him!** If you have friends and family members, neighbors and work colleagues who are still held captive by addiction and unbelief, you have at least one clear calling on your life today: share your faith by sharing your transformed life with them. Share your faith out loud, right where you are today.

God, I'm not very smart, but I have a "here I am, send me" heart. So You've got to make it clear, Lord. You've just got to! Tell me what You want me to do and I'll do it. But please, please don't make it hard for me to understand because my heart's desire is to do Your will. In Jesus's clarifying name, Amen.

day 36

TWO MASTERS

No one can serve two masters. Either you will hate the one and love the other, or you will be devoted to the one and despise the other. You cannot serve both God and money.

Matthew 6:24 NIV

WE HAVE A HARD TIME fixing our eyes on Jesus when we're fixated on food, running to the pantry when we could be running after Him. We simply can't run in two different directions at the same time. When we spend our lives pursuing one thing, it often means we're choosing to run away from something or someone else. The Message translates Matthew 6:24 this way, "You can't worship two gods at once. Loving one god, you'll end up hating the other. Adoration of one feeds contempt for the other. You can't worship God and Money both."

Likely, you picked up this book and began to fast and pray because you were convicted that sugar had an unhealthy hold on you. Not only was it ruining your health but it had moved from a physical stronghold to a spiritual one. Sugar had become master and you had become slave.

Sometimes I feel like Esau. In Genesis 25, this biblical figure was so hungry that he sold his birthright for a bowl of lentil stew and some bread. It sounds crazy that Esau allowed hunger to hold so much power over his life that it dictated his future, but I know I've let my appetite make decisions for me in the past. I don't know about a bowl of lentil stew, but I know I've traded God's best for me in exchange for a bowl of . . . ice cream with extra hot fudge.

God's Word is clear: You can't serve two masters at once! If sugar has made you its slave, perhaps it's time to tell sugar to take a hike. Christ came to set you free from all the other masters, leaving Himself as the one true and trustworthy guardian of your life. When something other than Christ has mastery over your life, it's easy to forget the Master.

When something other than Christ has mastery over your life, it's easy to forget the Master.

Perhaps it's not sugar that has a firm grip on you. Maybe it's money. The accumulation of money, the spending of money, the perception of having money—it dictates the car you drive, the friends you have over for dinner, the neighborhood you live in, the clothes you wear, the things you talk about in line at the grocery store, and the pictures you share online. Making money rules your thought life; spending money even more so. Maybe it's to the point that you can't go to Target to pick up a tube of toothpaste and a box of Ziploc baggies without spending fifty dollars on everything else that catches your eye. When you're ruled by something other than the Spirit, you are unruly, undisciplined, and out of control. You lack the spiritual fruit of self-control—in your eating, your spending, and your time online.

Or perhaps your master is your phone. It bosses you around each time it rings and you come running. It buzzes and you get an extra shot of dopamine, making your heart soar. You get a notification that someone liked what you said on social media, so you forget and forego the flesh-and-blood people right in front of you, the ones that God has charged you with loving (not merely liking).

You can't serve two masters. It's time to make a clear-cut choice.

> If you decide for God, living a life of God-worship, it follows that you don't fuss about what's on the table at mealtimes or whether the clothes in your closet are in fashion. There is far more to your life than the food you put in your stomach, more to your outer appearance than the clothes you hang on your body. Look at the birds, free and unfettered, not tied down to a job description, careless in the care of God. And you count far more to him than birds. (Matt. 6:25–26 MSG)

Where are you spending your life—your hours and your calories and your heart-affection?

This isn't to say that anything you do apart from spending time in prayer and reading the Bible is wrong. No, not at all! But you have to look back to the greatest commandment of all: "You shall love the LORD your God with all your heart and with all your soul and with all your might" (Deut. 6:5). When you

Jesus is the only master that gives freedom to those who are bound to Him.

love Him first and foremost, you invest your attention and affection in a high-yielding fund. The account increases and compounds so that you might enjoy all the other gifts that your master has blessed you with as well. But when you spend your affection and attention on the other masters who tempt you, you come to the true Master bankrupt—broke and broken. This isn't the first time you've heard me say this.

Jesus is the only master that gives freedom to those who are bound to Him. Being a slave to anything else simply leaves you tangled up.

Master Jesus, You are the one and only good God. Be master of my heart and master of my days. Master over my eating and my spending. I come to You, fully submitted to Your lordship over my life, because You alone are Lord. There is none beside You. With the ongoing help of Your Spirit, I refuse to let any false masters boss me around again. I'm convicted and convinced that You're the only master who loves me, who leads me, who laid down His life for me. Only You, Master Jesus! Thank You and Amen.

day 37

KEEP KNOCKING,
KEEP ASKING

Ask and keep on asking and it will be given to you; seek and keep
on seeking and you will find; knock and keep on knocking and
the door will be opened to you.

Matthew 7:7 AMP

SOMETIMES MEN AND WOMEN who fast with me come
to the end of their forty days and cry out, "Where are the miracles? Where is the gentle whisper? And why do I still want
to lick all the frosting off of all the cupcakes in all the world?"

I love how the Amplified translation of the Bible explains
exactly how we are to ask for and seek the Lord: persistently
persistent. Over and over again we are to ask God to set us free,
to speak to our hearts, to convict and transform us. Tirelessly,
we are to pray for those we know and love. Though we grow
weary of crying out and calling out, this is how we are to ask
for healing from the Great Physician and good blessings from
the Giver of all good gifts. Over and over and over again. "Ask
and keep on asking and it will be given to you; seek *and* keep on

seeking and you will find; knock *and* keep on knocking and the door will be opened to you" (Matt. 7:7 AMP, emphasis added).

God hasn't invited us to a one-and-done type of conversation. He's inviting us to a "pray without ceasing" (1 Thess. 5:17) sort of dialogue. An eternal back and forth. If there are things that you hoped to hear and receive from the Lord during this fast but haven't yet, keep asking. Keep knocking. Keep seeking.

Jesus was so committed to teaching us this persistently persistent method of prayer, He illustrated it in a parable. The parable of the persistent widow, found in Luke 18:1–8, paints a picture of a woman who pleaded for help before a judge who didn't fear God or care about the needs of others. Over and over again, day in and day out, the widow returned to the judge, begging for his help. Eventually the selfish judge agreed to help her, not because he loved her but because he loved his own peace and quiet.

Perhaps you've heard the term "the squeaky wheel gets the grease." The judge wanted the widow to stop squeaking, to stop pestering him. How much more will the eternal Judge, the Father of our Lord Jesus Christ, respond to your persistent prayers, for He loves you beyond measure.

One of my earliest memories as a new mom took place late one night as I nursed my infant son in the rocking chair beside his crib. In the dimly lit nursery, I opened up my Bible and turned to Matthew 7. "Ask and it will be given to you," I read, "seek and you will find; knock and the door will be opened to you. For everyone who asks receives; the one who seeks finds; and to the one who knocks, the door will be opened" (vv. 7–8 NIV). Though I was familiar with the passage, the words that followed felt brand-new in light of the baby in my arms. I continued reading. "Which of you, if your son asks for bread, will give him a stone? Or if he asks for a fish, will give him a snake?

If you, then, though you are evil, know how to give good gifts to your children, how much more will your Father in heaven give good gifts to those who ask him!" (Matt. 7:9–11 NIV). Though I still love that baby who is now a teenager, I realize I am more like the unjust judge in the parable than I am like our generous God. I want to be generous, but selfish motives often taint my responses, even to my kids. God the Father, however, is untainted. He responds to our every prayer with pure love.

God is not like us. His love transcends selfishness and surpasses the nursing mother's tender adoration. Because His ear is inclined toward us perpetually, we can pray persistently. He doesn't grow weary of our sin-struggles the way we grow weary of our own children's challenges. The way we grow weary when they toddle to us morning, noon, and night with the same questions. God never gives up or gives in to selfishness and pride. He loves it when we come to Him as both Father and Judge.

> *Because His ear is inclined toward us perpetually, we can pray persistently.*

If you have prayed and sought the Lord as you fasted only to hear radio silence on the other end of the line, here are three things you could try.

1. **Ask God to inspire your prayers.** Ask Him to give you clarity in what to pray. Sometimes I ask God, *Lord, show me what You're doing in my life (or in my children's lives or my spouse's life) so that I might prayerfully and purposefully join You there.* Asking God what to pray may seem backward, but it has brought a beautiful order to my prayer life. God is your kind and generous Father; He longs to give you every good gift, so ask Him what He has in store for you. Perhaps, here in these last few

KEEP KNOCKING, KEEP ASKING **191**

days, you will find yourself praying an entirely different sort of prayer. If He puts something new on your heart, obey and pray.

2. **Pray like a squeaky wheel.** Morning and noon and nighttime too, talk to the Lord about your needs and the needs of others. Remind Him of the prayers He inspired you to pray, and confess your trust in Him out loud, again and again. And when you are tempted to doubt that He's listening or that He will answer your requests, remind Him of His Word, *God, You've told me, "You do not have because you do not ask"* (James 4:2 NIV). *Well, here I am asking.* Then set the alarm on your phone to remind you to pray it again tomorrow.

3. **Trust God for the timing and don't stop asking.** It is possible that your prayers on a certain matter may not be answered for some time yet. If that is the case, but you feel the Spirit prompting you that you are praying in accordance with God's will, don't stop praying. Just because you're drawing near to the end of your fast doesn't mean you've laid down your final Amen. It's possible that this prayer will be an anthem prayer, something you pray for a very long time. Asking God to heal your marriage, asking Him to pursue your prodigal child and bring him or her home to faith again, asking God for physical healing and emotional healing too . . . the Lord deals with some of these prayers over time, so don't stop bringing your concerns before Him.

> *Just because you're drawing near to the end of your fast doesn't mean you've laid down your final Amen.*

As Matthew 7:7 instructs, continue to "ask *and* keep on asking . . . seek *and* keep on seeking . . . knock *and* keep on knocking" (AMP). The door will be opened to you if it's the door God knows is best. Just ask and keep on asking. Because His ear is inclined toward us perpetually, we can pray persistently.

Heavenly Father, thank You for never giving up. Thank You for being a good, gift-giving dad. Thank You for giving me the strength to keep praying and keep trusting and keep clinging to Your goodness. In Jesus's enduring and endurance-strengthening name, Amen.

day 38

GETTING DOWN
TO THE ROOT

Blessed is the one
    who does not walk in step with the wicked
or stand in the way that sinners take
    or sit in the company of mockers,
but whose delight is in the law of the LORD,
    and who meditates on his law day and night.
That person is like a tree planted by streams of
    water,
    which yields its fruit in season
and whose leaf does not wither—
    whatever they do prospers.

Not so the wicked!
    They are like chaff
    that the wind blows away.

Psalm 1:1–4 NIV

THIS PAST MONTH, my youngest son has been learning about the water cycle in his science class. One interesting way that water is syphoned up from the ground is with the help of trees. Transpiration is the process by which root systems drink up groundwater, carry the water up the trunk, through the branches, and finally out to the green leaves where the moisture exits the plant in the form of water vapor. Warm air lifts the water vapor up into the sky until the temperatures cool and water droplets form around tiny dust particles. Millions of minuscule drops gather together to create a cloud. When the cloud gets heavy enough, water drops in the form of precipitation, nourishing the earth once again.

Oftentimes I look around at the natural world and am overcome by the reality of a creative Creator who so lovingly provides all we need. Good, pure, life-giving water. Yet sometimes I choose to drink from the wrong source, gulping down polluted lies that lead to a polluted life.

Psalm 1 has been one of my favorite Bible passages for most of my life. I love the imagery of a flourishing tree that starts down at the root system. It is both poetic and practical, beautiful and biological. Just like a tree, when the roots of our lives reach down deep and tap into a healthy water source, we thrive and bear fruit, season after season. But not any old water will do.

If you want a flourishing life, you must abide beside nourishing streams. Similarly, if you want to bear the fruit of God's Spirit in your thought life, your thoughts must be rooted in His Word. If you want your work life and your eating life and your home life to bear the right kind of fruit, you must be firmly planted by the right kind of water. Before you can embrace a healthy life, expecting health to extend its branches out beyond these forty days, you must consider where you have been rooted all these years. Addictions

If you want a flourishing life, you must abide beside nourishing streams.

don't spring up by accident, you know. Addictions grow on the branches of lives that are rooted beside the wrong water source.

Earlier we talked about some of our food triggers, those age-old habits and hurts that cause us to run to food or drink for comfort or reward. Of course, to plant our lives beside life-giving streams, we must first uproot them from the rancid flow of lies we've believed in the past. **Just as truth nourishes healthy lives, lies feed unhealthy lives.**

Take a moment to pinpoint the lies from which your roots have been drinking. Perhaps you've been overweight since early childhood, and you drink these words daily: "Nothing I do has ever changed my weight or my eating. Nothing ever will." If you are planted beside this lie, you've got to yank it out by the root and replant your life beside what is scripturally true: "God's Word says that He makes all things new. I am loved by the Lord who came to set prisoners free and heal those who are sick. I am ready for God to do a new thing in my life because He told me that He can and that He will!"

"Overeating makes me happy" is another familiar lie. Pull it out by the root and replant your life beside this truth instead: "The joy of the Lord is my strength. With Him I am overcome with joy. I don't want a dopamine-induced happiness that a sugar high brings. I want the satisfied joy that the Most High offers to those who are planted in His Word and in His presence."

If you have believed the lie that you are unloved and unlovable, pull it out and plant this in your heart: "I am eternally and abundantly loved."

Maybe the lies you've believed are now lies that you act upon. "I deserve a bowl of ice cream after a long day with the kids." "I deserve a candy bar from the checkout lane at the grocery

196 THE 40-DAY SUGAR FAST

store." "I deserve a win after a day of losses at work." Here's the truth you need to ingest today: You don't deserve anything. You can have it if you want it, but it's not your just desserts. As a matter of fact, when you live this reward-centered life, playing tit for tat with mochas and wine, your "reward" will end up feeling more like a curse.

I'm reminded of the lesson we learned on day 10: **God is our reward.** That's the truth we need to abide by. When we turn to our next sugar high instead of the Most High, we don't get lifted high. We end up feeling lower than before because, after a sugar high comes a sugar crash—and that's no reward at all. **When we turn to sugar-substitutes for our reward, we end up both physically and spiritually malnourished.**

You're coming to the end of these forty days of fasting from sugar, but I want to encourage you to fast from lies for the rest of your life. Uproot yourself from a negative inner dialogue, then plant yourself beside true waters. The way to plant yourself in the truth is to plant the truth in yourself. Combat the lies you hear with nourishing truth straight from the Bible. That's what Jesus did. When He was tempted by the devil during His forty-day fast in the wilderness, He fought back by speaking truth. Here's how it began:

The way to plant yourself in the truth is to plant the truth in yourself.

> Then Jesus was led up by the Spirit into the wilderness to be tempted by the devil. And after fasting forty days and forty nights, he was hungry. And the tempter came and said to him, "If you are the Son of God, command these stones to become loaves of bread." But he answered, "It is written,
>
> 'Man shall not live by bread alone,
>   but by every word that comes from the mouth of
>   God.'" (Matt. 4:1–4)

When you are firmly planted beside true waters, nourished by and meditating on God's Word, what you read becomes what you speak. What you take in flows out. It's the living water cycle!

Forty days of truth won't be enough to sustain you for life. This must become a lifestyle now. Whether you pick up a candy bar on day 41 or continue living a sugar-free life, continue feasting on the Bible! Ingest God's Word because that's where God has invested His transforming power!

Oh Lord, thank You for Your Word. Increase in me a hunger for it, because it brings nourishment to my life. As I meditate upon its truth, establish my roots so that I might drink deeply and bear Your fruit in my life. In Jesus's fruitful name, I pray, Amen.

day 39

GOD WANTS YOUR LIFE, NOT YOUR SUGAR

Therefore, I urge you, brothers and sisters, in view of God's mercy, to offer your bodies as a living sacrifice, holy and pleasing to God—this is your true and proper worship. Do not conform to the pattern of this world, but be transformed by the renewing of your mind. Then you will be able to test and approve what God's will is—his good, pleasing and perfect will.

Romans 12:1–2 NIV

THIS FAST WAS NEVER about the sugar. Remember, our sugar cravings were simply the doorway through which we invited the Holy Spirit into our hungry lives. Once He came in, He looked around, smiled, nodded, and said, "Thanks for the sugar, but I want it all."

God doesn't want your sugar; He wants your life. A physical detox isn't going to leave you changed. Forty days in the Word won't outweigh the other 325 you spend chasing the world this year. There's more to it than that. If all you did during your fast was surrender your sugar on the altar before the Lord, then you misunderstood the whole point. **God doesn't want a temporary sugar sacrifice; He wants a forever living sacrifice.**

Hudson Taylor, a missionary from the nineteenth century, once said, "Christ is either Lord of all, or He is not Lord at all."[1] We can't invite the Lord to inhabit our lives like a dwelling place, then ask Him to stay out of the small room at the end of the hall.

> *God doesn't want your sugar; He wants your life.*

He must be the sovereign ruler over our whole metaphorical home. That's why we keep coming back to consider if there's any "room" we need to surrender to His lordship in order to make more room for Him. Even now, in a humble, eleventh-hour attempt to invite the Lord to be Lord of all, let's read the passage above once more, considering a few key phrases.

In view of God's mercy. Don't skim over these four little words that appear near the beginning of Romans 12. In light of God's mercy—mercy simply means that He withholds His judgment so that we might know His grace—how should we live? In light of all He's done to rescue and redeem us, how can we help but love Him back? I'm not talking about just a little love; I'm talking about all our love. Not only has He given us each new day but He's also granted us an eternity of days in His kingdom of light. In light of that, we should respond with our whole selves. **We should give Him access to our whole lives because He saved our whole lives!**

Holy and pleasing to God—this is your true and proper worship. God is speaking directly to Christ followers here. He is saying: "Since I made you holy, live holy. Since I made you pleasing, be pleasing. This holy and pleasing life is how you worship Me. Your holy and pleasing life is an offering of thanks back to Me." Every moment of every day, with our lives set upon the altar, this is how we worship.

Do not conform to the pattern of this world. We know the temptation to conform to the world, rather than conform to the Word. With only two days left in our fast, we need to be sure to heed this warning or we'll end up right back where we started. Though we've experienced both physical and spiritual breakthroughs, the world is eager to get us back in its clutches and tangled in old, familiar sins. That's why we need to throw off anything and everything that hinders us as we transition into life beyond the fast.

> Therefore, since we are surrounded by such a great cloud of witnesses, let us throw off everything that hinders and the sin that so easily entangles. And let us run with perseverance the race marked out for us. (Heb. 12:1 NIV)

You're enlisted in God's service now. Second Timothy 2:4 says, "No soldier in active service entangles himself in the affairs of everyday life, so that he may please the one who enlisted him as a soldier" (NASB). Don't get tied up with the affairs of everyday life again. Whether you choose to remain sugar-free or not, you must continue to live free!

Transition out of this fast carefully, so that you don't find yourself running back to sugar instead of God. **If you give the devil a foothold, sugar may become a stronghold again.** Test and approve God's will for your life carefully.

If you aren't sure what God's will for you is beyond this fast, keep spending time with Him. Stay in His Word and pray. Focus your thinking on God's will, and He will transform your thinking to match His will. If you let Him, God will renew your mind so that you might clearly understand His will—His good, pleasing, and perfect will. You've simply got to stay close to Him. All of you placed on the altar before Him. I love how the Message implores us:

So here's what I want you to do, God helping you: Take your everyday, ordinary life—your sleeping, eating, going-to-work, and walking-around life—and place it before God as an offering. Embracing what God does for you is the best thing you can do for him. Don't become so well-adjusted to your culture that you fit into it without even thinking. Instead, fix your attention on God. You'll be changed from the inside out. Readily recognize what he wants from you, and quickly respond to it. Unlike the culture around you, always dragging you down to its level of immaturity, God brings the best out of you, develops well-formed maturity in you. (Rom. 12:1–2)

That's what this fast has been about all about. Staying close to Jesus! **He never wanted your sugar, it's you He's been after all along.**

Dear Lord, You can have it all. You can have my waking and my sleeping, my holidays and my ordinary days too. You can have my weekdays and my weekends, my daytime and my nighttime. You can have my thinking and my feeling too. Take my sugar and take my life. You, God, can have it all! Amen.

NEARING THE END

As you near the end of your fast, let me encourage you to see the end as a beginning. This intimate fasting friendship doesn't have to be reserved for times when you need a spiritual breakthrough. Now that you know how tangible, how present, how very wonderfully near God is, make fasting a regular part of your relationship with Him.

After five years of doing these forty-day sugar fasts, I decided to try a new type of fasting. Today I fast during the morning hours Monday through Friday and break my fast at noon. My time in the

Word has never been more applicable; my time in prayer, never more conversational; and my sensitivity to the promptings of the Spirit, never more exciting.

Instead of setting aside a season to fast, choose seasons *not* to fast. Take breaks from the intimate practice of fasting in order to spend more time enjoying the things of this world—rather than the other way around. When friends are in town or the holidays are upon us or you're traveling, fast from fasting. As you near the end of these forty days, consider the benefits of this fast and how you might continue to enjoy the feasting life!

day 40

LIVE LIKE IT'S TRUE!

Satisfy us in the morning with your unfailing love,
that we may sing for joy and be glad all our days.

Psalm 90:14 NIV

LONG-TERM HUNGER can leave a long and lasting mark on a person. My grandparents, who were raised during the Great Depression, never wasted food or money. They always took their leftovers home from restaurants. Grandma kept an account of every grocery item she bought. After she died, I came across a pile of spiral notebooks that listed every purchase, every box of powdered milk and each five-cent stick of gum. She used each tea bag multiple times and taught me to do the same. Growing up hungry marked the way she shopped, cooked, ate, saved, and lived.

Growing up hungry left a mark on me as well, only mine was a different kind of hunger. For the first twenty-five years of my life, I experienced an emotional hunger that drove me to food and the approval of others. That's how old I was when I finally came across the verse above and committed it to memory. I decided that bondage-breaking day to pray Psalm 90:14 every morning, believing that Christ was the only One who was able to satiate my hungry heart. I told Him that I was willing to cry out morning after morning, but He had to do the filling. After all, He made my heart; He knew every crack and crevice, every hurt and every hole.

I had come to a point in my life, and perhaps you have too, where no person or purchase, not even a half-baked pan of brownies, could fill me up. I was at the end of trying because I'd tried it all. After twenty-five years, I gave God complete access to my hungry heart, much more of me than I had given Him before. I prayed, *Lord, satisfy me with your unfailing love this morning so that I may sing for joy and be glad all day long.*

While I was eager for an instant filling that would keep me supernaturally satiated until bedtime, it was more complicated than that. As I said, long-term hunger leaves its mark. So I made a choice to believe that God had, indeed, faithfully filled me that morning, instantaneously and supernaturally, whether I felt it or not. I had to learn to live satisfied. I was accustomed to feeling hungry and running to food. I needed to learn to live differently, because my life was now different. This new awareness of having been made full had to reshape my thinking, one believing moment at a time.

Throughout those early days especially, when loneliness or insecurities threatened me, I had to recognize the lies and actively decide that they were false. "I'm not hungry, I'm full," I'd say to myself. "I'm not insecure; I am completely secure as a child of the One who filled me up this morning. I'm full, and I'm glad I'm full." My inner dialogue throughout the day worked to keep me in step with God's answered prayer every morning.

The key to living a full life beyond this fast is actively reminding yourself that you have been filled. Choose to believe that God has filled you, and then live like it's true! Believe that you are full, and you will live a full life. Keep believing it and keep walking it out each day.

So often, at the end of these forty days, I hear this question: "How do I stop myself from falling right back into my sugar addiction again?" My answer is simply, "Keep in step with what is true, and keep in step with the Spirit!" **As you step beyond this fast, remember the truth of God's filling, or you will run to false fillers again.**

Believe that you are full, and you will live a full life.

Today I want to serve up one final helping of Scripture. Read slowly, savoring one of our final meals together. As you read, look for specific instructions to help you stay the course in the days ahead.

> It is for freedom that Christ has set us free. Stand firm, then, and do not let yourselves be burdened again by a yoke of slavery. . . .
>
> So I say, walk by the Spirit, and you will not gratify the desires of the flesh. For the flesh desires what is contrary to the Spirit, and the Spirit what is contrary to the flesh. They are in conflict with each other, so that you are not to do whatever you want. But if you are led by the Spirit, you are not under the law.
>
> The acts of the flesh are obvious: sexual immorality, impurity and debauchery; idolatry and witchcraft; hatred, discord, jealousy, fits of rage, selfish ambition, dissensions, factions and envy; drunkenness, orgies, and the like. I warn you, as I did before, that those who live like this will not inherit the kingdom of God.
>
> But the fruit of the Spirit is love, joy, peace, forbearance, kindness, goodness, faithfulness, gentleness and self-control. Against such things there is no law. Those who belong to Christ Jesus have crucified the flesh with its passions and desires. Since we live by the Spirit, let us keep in step with the Spirit. (Gal. 5:1, 16–25 NIV)

My fasting friends, it is for a life of freedom that Christ set you free. The Spirit of God, which you have been consuming, is calling you to stand against the pull of the flesh. Follow His lead and stand firm by His side. Stay the course, whether He leads you to remain sugar-free or not.

Stay close to God and you won't go running after false gods again. Stay close to God and you won't go running after false gods again. Fill your life with the Spirit, and you won't indulge the flesh. Live each day in the truth of Psalm 90:14: God has filled you with Himself.

It is true that a long life of hunger leaves an impression, but a satisfied life leaves a lasting mark too. Live like it's true!

Dear Lord, let this fast leave a lasting mark on me. You have satisfied me with Yourself, and I am full. Help me, Holy Spirit, to keep in step with the knowledge of my satisfied, Spirit-filled life, so that I do not turn again to the temporary fillers that deaden my hunger for You. Keep me hungry, Lord, so that I might daily know that You have made me full. Thank You for these forty days. In Jesus's name, Amen.

WELL DONE!

Congratulations on reaching the end of the 40-Day Sugar Fast! I have one more chapter for you to gobble up tomorrow, because I don't want you to stop feasting just because you're done fasting. Don't forget to celebrate by heading over to 40daysugarfast.com. Find the video entitled "Life beyond the fast," where I offer encouragement on how to remain free, even if you don't remain sugar-free! Then click over to the testimonials page where you can leave me a note. I'd love to hear from you!

day 41

HE'S NOT DONE
WITH YOU YET

Like newborn babies, crave pure spiritual milk, so that by it you may grow up in your salvation, now that you have tasted that the Lord is good.

1 Peter 2:2–3 NIV

SURPRISE! You thought you were done, but you're never really done! You've officially completed your forty-day fast, but now you have some choices to make about the life laid out before you. How will you live it? Whatever you feed regularly will grow throughout your life. Feed your belly, and it will grow. Feed the spirit, and it will grow. Feed your earthly cravings, and they will grow. But feed your spiritual cravings every day, and they will grow abundantly, exceedingly more than forty days can capture. What will you feed on today and tomorrow and the next day and the next? Will you run back to the things that tempted you in the past or will you continue to chase hard after God? You get to make a new plan because this is a new life. The slate is clean and your palate is too.

Your body is strong and healthy and your mind is alert. How will you live? The choice is yours.

The One who brought down each stronghold in your life is inviting you to continue enjoying His strong hold.

The same God who brought down the figurative walls of Jericho in your life, the walls that held you back, is calling you to grow up and enter into the life that He has prepared for you. The One who brought down each stronghold in your life is inviting you to continue enjoying His strong hold.

"Like newborn babies, crave pure spiritual milk, so that by it you may grow up in your salvation" (1 Pet. 2:2 NIV). **The God who called you to salvation is charging you now to grow up and continue working out your salvation.**

> Therefore, my dear friends, as you have always obeyed—not only in my presence, but now much more in my absence—continue to work out your salvation with fear and trembling. (Phil. 2:12 NIV)

You don't need me to lead you another day! You've got the Word of God at your fingertips and the Holy Spirit camped within you. No, you don't need me. You've tasted freedom in Him, and you know that He is enough for you. This transition reminds me of King Josiah and the children of Israel, and how Josiah helped God's people hear the Word of the Lord. Once they committed to obeying God's Word as a nation, the king brought down all the high places that the previous generations had erected to false gods. The Israelites followed their leader, and an entire people turned their faces to the Lord together. However, after Josiah died, a new king took the throne and eventually the people turned back to their sinful ways. Up went their idols and before long they found themselves in bondage once again.

In a way, I took the role of Josiah these last forty days, inviting you to tear down the false idols by denying the false fillers in your life. Today I'm leaving you to continue on without me. My job here is through. That's why I'm urging you to commit to following the true King in the days to come. You don't need this guide. Christ Himself has left you with a guide, His Holy Spirit, and a light to illuminate your path, His Holy Word.

I have led you through your personal exodus from sugar captivity into the promised land of health and wholeness. Now you must go on without me. Keep walking it out, one step at a time, one hard day at a time, one tempting meal at a time, one applicable passage of Scripture at a time. Each time you're tempted to run to the pantry, run to Jesus. Run to Jesus when you believe that only a glass of wine can help you cope. Turn to His holy face, rather than turning to Facebook.

What God is offering you now is a complete makeover, a forever transformation! That's why you must continue to grow up and mature in your faith. **God's not done with you yet.** Now that those sugar shackles have fallen from your wrists, press on in your freedom and work it *God's not done* out 365 days of the year. Don't stop. *with you yet.*

"For I am confident of this very thing, that He who began a good work in you will perfect it until the day of Christ Jesus" (Phil. 1:6 NASB). Praise God for His ongoing commitment to you, but hear this: Since He is committed to you, you must also be committed to you! Of course, God should be your first priority, but you need to value yourself because He values you. You must value your freedom, both externally and internally, presently and forevermore, for it was bought with the precious blood of Christ.

On day 41, the best way to value your life is by consuming more and more of that good-for-you spiritual milk! You're craving it now . . . keep craving it.

Break the fast if you wish, but don't stop feasting. The feasting life is the sweetest life!

Dear Lord, I want to live free. I do not want to get tangled up in old sins again. Holy Spirit, abide in me as I abide in You, so that I might bear the fruit of self-control in my life. I know that's an important part of not getting entangled again. Thank You for filling my belly and filling my mind and filling my life with pure spiritual milk these past forty-one days. I am committed to following You on day 42 and day 43 and day 44 and day 45 . . . because You have set me free! Thank You. Amen.

APPENDIX A

LIFE BEYOND THE FAST

YOU ARE FREE! Now the choice is yours if you want to remain sugar-free. God's Word says that everything is permissible, but not everything is beneficial. Perhaps you've found that refined sugar simply isn't good for you. You lost weight and found energy and clarity. Your joint pain and bellyaches are gone, and your sleep is better than it has been for decades. Your relationships are better too, because you're not riding a sugar coaster up and down each afternoon. Just because you *can* eat sugar doesn't mean that you *should*.

Here are five practical ideas for how to limit your sugar year-round so that you can feel physically healthy, emotionally stable, and spiritually alert.

1. **Make your sugar fast a sugar-free lifestyle.** Perhaps you want to go sugar-free forever, but you also want to be able to cheat every now and then. Here's the trick: Instead of taking a break from your highly sugared life, think of those "cheats" as little breaks from a sugar-free lifestyle. Live sugar-free but don't be afraid to fast from

your sugar fast every now and again. Do you see how it's practically the same thing—just backwards? Instead of taking breaks from sugar to detox, live clean and clear and free from sugar most of the time, then take breaks when there's a special occasion that includes a special treat.

2. **Never eat alone.** My most unhealthy eating choices have taken place when I've been alone. A few years ago I made the choice to only eat special treats in the company of family and friends. (And it's usually been for family and friends and fun events that I've made a batch of lemon bars or a cheesecake!) Even when I take the baked goods out of the oven and cut them up to place upon a platter, I don't nibble on crumbled edges until I'm with my loved ones. It's one way I love myself. I'm keeping in step with the Spirit as I practice self-control. (If you struggle with drinking alcohol daily, this is a good boundary for you too. Never drink alone. Never eat alone.)

3. **Give your leftovers away!** If you follow the second guideline, then this one should be easy! Package up any leftover cookies and cake and send them home as a gift to your loved ones. If you're baking for your little family, put leftovers in the freezer or walk a plate of cookies over to a neighbor.

4. **Discover wonderful sugar-free treats.** During the fast, I warned you not to exchange one obsession for another; however, if you want to make this low-sugar lifestyle manageable year-round, now's a good time to discover some sweet treats that are sugar-free. For a list of my favorite sugar-free recipes, visit 40daysugar fast.com.

5. **Join me again next year.** Finally, make the 40-Day
   Sugar Fast an annual event, and invite your family and
   friends to join you. You can link up with me every January at 40daysugarfast.com. Even when I'm actively
   living sugar-free, this annual fast works like a charm,
   reminding me to hunger and thirst for the satisfying
   sweetness of my Savior once again!

APPENDIX B

ADDITIONAL RESOURCES

THIS BOOK DOESN'T FOCUS on what is happening physiologically as you fast. I don't list the scientific reasons why you're addicted to sugar, and I don't offer sugar-free solutions. My single purpose is to lead you straight into the satisfying presence of the sweet Savior Himself. He's the missing ingredient, and the recipe to living the full life.

If, however, you would like to understand what is happening in your body as you detox, more information about why we crave sugar so intensely, and what that has to do with your spiritual life, here are a few of my favorite resources.

- *The Case Against Sugar* by Gary Taubes is a convincing look at both the addictive and destructive qualities of sugar. This is a great resource for those who are struggling with diabetes. Likewise, *Suicide by Sugar* by Nancy Appleton and G. N. Jacobs links our sugar intake to even more of our nation's health epidemics, from dementia to obesity to cancer.

- *Full: Food, Jesus, and the Battle For Satisfaction* by Asheritah Ciuciu offers an honest look at food fixation while pointing readers to the only One who can satisfy. And Asheritah's book *Bible and Breakfast: 31 Mornings with Jesus* couples sugar-free breakfast recipes with a short, easy-to-consume morning Bible study. *Bible and Breakfast* would be a wonderful resource to use during the transition into post-fast life.

- *Made to Crave: Satisfying Your Deepest Desire with God, Not Food* by Lysa TerKeurst reminds us that God created us to crave Him. This book serves as a reminder that, too often, our cravings are misplaced and misunderstood.

- *The Whole30: The 30-Day Guide to Total Health and Food Freedom* by Melissa and Dallas Hartwig is more than a recipe book; it's a movement! Hundreds of thousands of people have followed her plan to experience radical physical and emotional benefits while eating whole foods.

- *The 21-Day Sugar Detox: Bust Sugar and Carb Cravings Naturally* by Diane Sanfilippo is another whole foods–based eating plan that works to reset the body with new, healthier, sugar-free habits.

Acknowledgments

Matt Brunner—Thank you for supporting me in both prayerful and practical ways each time I lead this fast online. Balancing loving you and the boys as I love on others (via books) isn't easy. I am so grateful for your willingness to share God's love by sharing your time with me.

Bill Jensen—Your partnership, wisdom, and affirmation are gifts to me. Matt and I both appreciate you so much.

Rebekah Guzman, Mark Rice, Wendy Wetzel, and the rest of the brilliant Baker team—You caught the vision and joined me in this sugar-free adventure! I pray that the Lord does exceedingly, abundantly more than all you hope or imagine with this book.

Liz Heaney—I prayed for an editor who would challenge me to be a better writer. Thank you for being God's answer to that prayer.

Alle McCloskey—For all the years you supported me online and behind the scenes, thank you.

Caleb Peavey and the Unmutable team—I'm so grateful that Baker said yes to bringing you on board *The 40-Day Sugar Fast* team. Thank you for enabling me to serve so many men and women around the world.

Asheritah Ciuciu—You've been my partner in this nearly from the start. How kind of the Lord to give us one another.

Angie Mosteller, Kelli Stuart, Bethany Hockenbury, Amber Rogers, and Michelle Sit—Your availability to read all the words and pray all the prayers never ceases to amaze me. Your serving me allows me to serve others better.

Christy Nueman, Jennifer McClure, Amy J. Bennett, Katie M. Reid, Monica Swanson, Alexis MacPhee, Christie Thomas, Amber Lia, Christin Slade, Kasia Gilbert, Becky Keife, Elisa Pullium, Sarah Leach, Sarah Bragg, Jane Manka, Julie Kieras, and so many others—Thank you for partnering with me over the years. I could not have done these annual online fasts without a team of hungry-for-Jesus women!

Notes

Foreword

1. John Piper, *A Hunger for God: Desiring God through Fasting and Prayer* (Wheaton: Crossway Books, 1997), 23.

Day 3 When Sugar Walls Crumble

1. John H. Sammis, "Trust and Obey," 1887.

Day 4 Trusting God with the Battle

1. Jennifer Regan, "Not So Sweet–The Average American Consumes 150-170 Pounds Of Sugar Each Year," *BambooCore*, https://Bamboocorefitness.com/not-so -sweet-the-average-american-consumes-150-170-pounds-of-sugar-each-year/.

Day 12 Food Triggers

1. "Eating Disorders," *National Institute of Mental Health*, https://www.nimh .nih.gov/health/topics/eating-disorders/index.shtml.
2. Dr. William Davis, "Wheat is an Opiate," *WheatBelly Blog*, April 17, 2012, https://www.wheatbellyblog.com/2012/04/wheat-is-an-opiate/.
3. Asheritah Ciuciu, *Full: Food, Jesus, and the Battle for Satisfaction* (Chicago: Moody Publishers, 2017), 140.

Day 14 What Else Are You Craving?

1. "Andrew Bonar Quotes," *Christian Quotes*, accessed January 18, 2019, https://www.christianquotes.info/quotes-by-author/andrew-bonar-quotes/.
2. The translation and corresponding information came from *BibleHub*, accessed May 31, 2019, https://biblehub.com/greek/2836.htm.
3. Blaise Pascal, *Pensées VII* (425)1670, Blaise Pascal, Pensées.
4. William Bright, *Jesus and the Intellectual* (San Bernardino, CA: Campus Crusade for Christ International, 1968).
5. Lysa TerKeurst, *Made to Crave Devotional: 60 Days to Craving God, Not Food* (Grand Rapids: Thomas Nelson, 2011), 39.

Day 17 Be Quiet and Be Transformed

1. Bob Sorge, *Secrets of the Secret Place* (Kansas City, MO: Oasis House, 2001), 11.
2. Sorge, *Secrets of the Secret Place*, 11.

Day 19 Have a Sober Mind

1. "The Alcohol Manifesto," *Whole9*, https://www.whole9life.com/2012/09/the-alcohol-manifesto.

Day 20 The World's Goods Aren't as Good

1. "Pierre Teilhard de Chardin Quotes," *BrainyQuote*, accessed January 18, 2019, https://www.brainyquote.com/authors/pierre_teilhard_de_chardi.

Day 22 Spiritual and Mental Clarity

1. Dennis Lee and Daniel Lee Kulick, "Omega-3 Fatty Acids Benefits, Uses, and List of Foods," *MedicineNet*, October 2, 2017, https://www.medicinenet.com/omega-3_fatty_acids/article.htm#what_are_omega-3_fatty_acids.

Day 23 Hunger Pangs

1. Bill Gaultiere, "Hungry Heart Scriptures," *Soul Shepherding*, July 23, 2006, https://www.soulshepherding.org/hungry-heart-scriptures.

Day 24 Healing Past Hurts

1. Rebecca K. Reynolds, "Sugar because I'm tired," Facebook, January 19, 2019, https:/www.facebook.com/permalink.php?story_fbid=2315071788725433&id=1619110878321531.

Day 28 Feed My Sheep

1. To learn more about sponsoring a child through Compassion International, visit https://www.compassion.com.
2. To learn more about supporting The LuLuTree, visit https://www.thelulutree.com/partner.

Day 32 Wake Up!

1. "Leonard Ravenhill Quotes," *GoodReads*, accessed January 18, 2019, https://www.goodreads.com/quotes/8298551.

Day 39 God Wants Your Life, Not Your Sugar

1. "27 Hudson Taylor Quotes," *Christian Quotes*, accessed March 14, 2019, https://www.christianquotes.info/quotes-by-author/hudson-taylor-quotes/#axzz5iARcOUlb.

Wendy Speake is a trained actress and heartfelt Bible teacher. During her career in Hollywood she longed to tell stories that point audiences to the Savior. Today she does just that: writing books and speaking at events where every Bible story and personal story leads people right into the presence of God.

Wendy lives in Southern California with her husband, Matt, and their three sons. She writes regularly about motherhood and leads Bible studies at WendySpeake.com. She is the coauthor of the popular parenting books *Triggers*, *Parenting Scripts*, and *Life Creative*.

Ready to Go —
D E E P E R ?

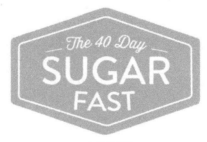

CONNECT WITH

Wendy

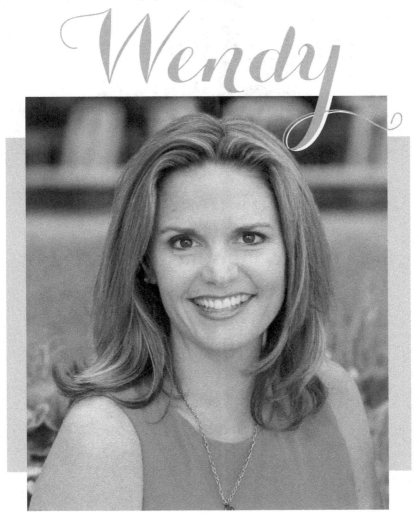

Discover more from Wendy at

WENDYSPEAKE.COM

or find her on Facebook or Instagram today.

 WendyJSpeake   wendy_speake

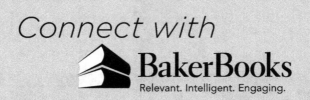
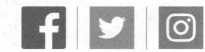